NURSING SERIES

Ambulatory Surgical Care

Second Edition

WESTERN® SCHOOLS

By
Nance A. Seiple, RN, CRNA, MEd

20 contact hours will be awarded upon successful completion of this course.
Western Schools is accredited as a provider of continuing nursing education by the American Nurses Credentialing Center's Commission on Accreditation.

P.O. Box 1930
Brockton, MA 02303
WESTERN SCHOOLS 1-800-438-8888

ABOUT THE AUTHOR

Nance A. Seiple, RN, CRNA, MEd, is an independent medical communications consultant based in suburban Chicago. A former nurse anesthesiology program director and staff member of the American Association of Nurse Anesthetists (AANA), she has extensive experience in the development and implementation of educational programs. Ms. Seiple received her MEd from the College of Education, Lehigh University. A member of the American Medical Writers Association and the National Association of Science Writers, Inc., her diverse publications include titles such as *Sedation and Analgesia for Outpatient Surgery* and *MRS to Treat Malignant Tumors*.

Nance Seiple has disclosed that she has no significant financial or other conflicts of interest pertaining to this course book.

ABOUT THE CONTENT EDITOR

Nancy Burden, MS, RN, CPAN, CAPA, is the director of ambulatory surgery for BayCare Health System in the Tampa Bay area of Florida. She holds two board certifications through the American Board of Perianesthesia Nursing Certification, Inc. She is a certified post anesthesia nurse (CPAN) and a certified ambulatory perianesthesia nurse (CAPA). Ms. Burden has written and edited numerous journal articles and book chapters on ambulatory surgery and perianesthesia nursing, including two editions of a major textbook on ambulatory surgical nursing. She is the editor for and currently sits on the editorial board of several publishers of perianesthesia and surgical-related journals. Ms. Burden also speaks nationally on a variety of topics related to ambulatory surgery. She is a member of the Association of Perioperative Registered Nurses (AORN), the Federated Ambulatory Surgery Association, and the American Association of Ambulatory Surgery Centers and serves as secretary of the Board of Directors for the Florida Society of Ambulatory Surgery Centers.

Nancy Burden has disclosed that she has no significant financial or other conflicts of interest pertaining to this course book.

Nurse Planner: Amy Bernard, MS, BSN, RN-BC

Amy Bernard has disclosed that she has no significant financial or other conflicts of interest pertaining to this course book.

Copy Editor: Liz Schaeffer

Indexer: Sylvia Coates

ISBN: 978-1-57801-306-7

P1011SH

COURSE INSTRUCTIONS

IMPORTANT: Read these instructions *BEFORE* proceeding!

COMPLETING THE FINAL EXAMINATION

Enclosed with your course book you will find a FasTrax® answer sheet. Use this answer sheet to respond to all the final exam questions that appear in this course. If the course has less than 100 questions, leave any remaining answer circles on the FasTrax answer sheet blank.

Be sure to fill in circles completely using **blue or black ink.** The FasTrax grading system will not read pencil. If you make an error, you may use correction fluid (such as White Out) to correct it.

FasTrax answer sheets are preprinted with your name and address and the course title. If you are completing more than one course, be sure to record your answers on the correct corresponding answer sheet.

A PASSING SCORE

The final exam is a multiple choice exam. You must score 70% or better in order to pass this course and receive a certificate of completion. Should you fail to achieve the required score, an additional FasTrax answer sheet will be sent to you so that you may make a second attempt to pass the course. You will be allowed three chances to pass the same course without incurring additional charges. After three failed attempts, your file will be closed.

RECORDING YOUR HOURS

Use the Study Time Log provided in this course book to monitor and record the time it takes to complete this course. Upon completion, tally your total time spent and use this information to respond to the final question of the course evaluation.

COURSE EVALUATIONS

The Course Evaluation provided in this course book is a critical component of the course and must be completed and submitted with your final exam. Responses to evaluation statements should be recorded in the lower right hand corner of the FasTrax answer sheet, in the section marked "Evaluation." Evaluations provide Western Schools with vital feedback regarding courses. Your feedback is important to us; please take a few minutes to complete the evaluation.

To provide additional feedback regarding this course, Western Schools services, or to suggest new course topics, use the space provided on the Important Information form found on the back of the FasTrax instruction sheet included with your course. Return the completed form to Western Schools with your final exam.

SUBMITTING THE COMPLETED FINAL EXAM

For your convenience, Western Schools provides a number of exam grading options. Full instructions and complete grading details are listed on the FasTrax instruction sheet provided with this course. If you are mailing your answer sheet(s) to Western Schools, we recommend you make a copy as a back-up.

COURSE COMPLETION TIME FRAMES AND EXTENSIONS

You have two (2) years from the date of purchase to complete this course. If you are not able to complete the course within 2 years, a six (6) month extension may be purchased. If you have not completed the course within 30 months from the original enrollment date, your file will be closed and no certificate will be issued.

CHANGE OF ADDRESS?

In the event that your address changes prior to completing this course, please call our customer service department at 1-800-618-1670, so that we may update your file.

WESTERN SCHOOLS GUARANTEES YOUR SATISFACTION

If any continuing education course fails to meet your expectations, or if you are not satisfied for any reason, you may return the course materials for an exchange or a refund (less shipping and handling) within 30 days. Software, video, and audio courses must be returned unopened. Textbooks must not be written in or marked up in any other way.

Thank you for using Western Schools to fulfill your continuing education needs!

WESTERN SCHOOLS
P.O. Box 1930
Brockton, MA 02303
(800) 438-8888
www.westernschools.com

WESTERN SCHOOLS
STUDY TIME LOG

AMBULATORY SURGICAL CARE

INSTRUCTIONS: Use this log sheet to document the amount of time you spend completing this course. Include the time it takes you to read the instructions, read the course book, take the final examination, and complete the evaluation.

Date	Time Spent Hours	Time Spent Minutes
____________	____________	____________
____________	____________	____________
____________	____________	____________
____________	____________	____________
____________	____________	____________
____________	____________	____________
____________	____________	____________
____________	____________	____________
____________	____________	____________
____________	____________	____________
____________	____________	____________
____________	____________	____________
____________	____________	____________
____________	____________	____________
____________	____________	____________
____________	____________	____________
TOTAL*	Hours	Minutes

*** Please use this total study time to answer the final question of the course evaluation.**

WESTERN SCHOOLS
COURSE EVALUATION

AMBULATORY SURGICAL CARE

INSTRUCTIONS: Using the scale below, please respond to the following evaluation statements. All responses should be recorded in the lower right-hand corner of the FasTrax answer sheet, in the section marked "Evaluation." Be sure to fill in each corresponding answer circle completely using blue or black ink. Leave any remaining answer circles blank.

A	B	C	D
Agree Strongly	Agree Somewhat	Disagree Somewhat	Disagree Strongly

OBJECTIVES: After completing this course, I am able to

1. Discuss how changes in the health care delivery system in the past century have influenced the utilization of ambulatory surgery.
2. Describe the selection of and preoperative assessment for the ambulatory surgical patient.
3. Recognize anesthetic agents and techniques and the applicability and appropriateness of each for ambulatory surgical procedures.
4. Discuss the role and responsibilities of the perioperative nurse in the care of patients receiving procedural sedation.
5. Identify the various aspects of nursing care needed for the safe transition of the patient from the immediate postoperative recovery phase to discharge from the facility.
6. Recognize serious complications and emergencies that may occur during ambulatory surgery and anesthesia.
7. Identify unique considerations relative to pediatric and geriatric populations in the ambulatory surgical setting.
8. Explain how patient safety, risk management, and quality improvement are integral parts of perioperative nursing practice.

COURSE CONTENT

9. The course materials were well-organized and clearly written.
10. The course expanded my knowledge and understanding of the subject matter.
11. This offering met my professional educational needs.
12. The final examination was well-written and at an appropriate level for the content of the course.

ATTESTATION

13. By submitting this answer sheet, I certify that I have read the course materials and personally completed the final examination based on the material presented. Mark "A" for Agree and "B" for Disagree.

COURSE HOURS

14. Please select the response that best reflects the total number of hours that it took to complete this **20-hour** course.

    A. More than 22 hours
    B. 18–22 hours
    C. 15–18 hours
    D. Fewer than 15 hours

Note: To provide additional feedback regarding this course, Western Schools services, or to suggest new course topics, use the space provided on the Important Information form found on the back of the FasTrax instruction sheet included with your course.

CONTENTS

FIGURES AND TABLES

PRETEST

1. Begin this course by taking the pretest. Circle the answers to the questions on this page, or write the answers on a separate sheet of paper. Do not log answers to the pretest questions on the FasTrax test sheet included with the course.
2. Compare your answers to the PRETEST KEY located at the end of the Pretest. The pretest key indicates the page where the content of that question is discussed. Make note of the questions you missed, so that you can focus on those areas as you complete the course.
3. Complete the course by reading the chapter and completing the exam questions at the end of the chapter. Answers to these exam questions should be logged on the FasTrax test sheet included with the course.

1. Currently, the deciding factor in determining where a surgical procedure will be performed is

   a. facility location.
   b. hospital affiliation.
   c. third-party reimbursement.
   d. facility reputation.

2. Ambulatory surgical patient care is especially challenging to the nurse because of the

   a. cost-containment measures.
   b. compressed time frame.
   c. care plans.
   d. complex admission forms.

3. The ambulatory surgical patient has a greater need for

   a. premedication.
   b. intraoperative monitoring.
   c. predischarge teaching.
   d. oral hydration.

4. A statement indicating the patient understands the nature of the surgery as well as the risks and benefits is considered

   a. due process.
   b. informed consent.
   c. Medicare compatible.
   d. facility specific.

5. Drugs that reduce or prevent vomiting are called

   a. antidiuretics.
   b. antibiotics.
   c. antianemics.
   d. antiemetics.

6. Adults generally undergo which type of anesthetic induction?

   a. Neuroleptic
   b. Inhalation
   c. Opioid
   d. Intravenous

7. The last phase of general anesthesia is

   a. induction.
   b. maintenance.
   c. delirium.
   d. emergence.

8. Hypotension is most likely to occur with

   a. brachial block.
   b. Bier block.
   c. spinal anesthesia.
   d. epidural anesthesia.

9. A professional atmosphere should be maintained during the procedure because of the possibility of the patient experiencing

   a. permanent paralysis.
   b. intraoperative pain.
   c. intraoperative awareness.
   d. retrograde amnesia.

10. Medical oxygen tanks containing nitrous oxide are colored

    a. blue.
    b. green.
    c. silver.
    d. grey.

11. In a sedated patient, the most frequent cause of airway obstruction is

    a. mucus.
    b. the tongue.
    c. foreign material.
    d. the epiglottis.

12. A sedated patient who cannot maintain an open airway may tolerate

    a. an oropharyngeal airway.
    b. a nasopharyngeal airway.
    c. a laryngeal airway.
    d. an endotracheal tube.

13. Hypotension in the postoperative patient may cause

    a. pain.
    b. nausea and vomiting.
    c. airway obstruction.
    d. agitation.

14. A parameter commonly used to assess patient readiness for discharge is

    a. memory testing.
    b. scoring criteria.
    c. nerve stimulation.
    d. passive resistance.

15. A commonly overlooked cause of nausea and vomiting is

    a. pain.
    b. opioids.
    c. shivering.
    d. benzodiazepines.

16. Dantrolene (Dantrium) is the specific pharmocologic agent for the treatment of

    a. postdural puncture headache.
    b. anaphylactic shock.
    c. aspiration pneumonitis.
    d. malignant hyperthermia.

17. Nerve damage in the legs is most likely to develop with the use of which surgical position?

   a. Prone
   b. Lithotomy
   c. Fowler's
   d. Left lateral

18. What is the weight of a 35-kg child in pounds?

   a. 77
   b. 70
   c. 60
   d. 55

19. Geriatric patients are prone to postoperative

   a. ventilatory problems.
   b. nausea.
   c. shivering.
   d. dizziness.

20. The difference between risk management and quality improvement is that risk management focuses on

   a. prevention of incidents or injuries.
   b. enhancemenet of standards of care.
   c. provision of health care.
   d. patterns of practice.

This concludes the pretest.

PRETEST KEY

1.	C	chapter 1
2.	B	chapter 1
3.	C	chapter 2
4.	B	chapter 2
5.	D	chapter 3
6.	D	chapter 3
7.	D	chapter 3
8.	C	chapter 3
9.	C	chapter 3
10.	A	chapter 3
11.	B	chapter 4
12.	B	chapter 4
13.	B	chapter 5
14.	B	chapter 5
15.	A	chapter 5
16.	D	chapter 6
17.	B	chapter 6
18.	A	chapter 7
19.	A	chapter 7
20.	A	chapter 8

INTRODUCTION

Ambulatory, also known as outpatient, same-day, or one-day surgery, allows the patient to return home on the day of the surgery. It is cost-effective for the patient, third-party payers, and government agencies. The patient is spared the stress and time commitment of hospitalization, usually benefits from a more rapid recovery period, and has a reduced risk of acquiring a hospital-related infection.

The concept has grown exponentially since the 1970s as a result of technological advances in surgery, anesthesia, expansion of managed care, changes in Medicare and Medicaid, and patient acceptance. This growth presents challenges and opportunities for nurses practicing in this demanding environment.

Skilled nursing care, based on sound principles, does not change with the location where the care is provided. Consequently, the intent of this course is not to review established principles of surgical nursing, but rather to address concerns, techniques, and innovations specific to the ambulatory surgical setting. It is especially directed to the nurse new to the specialty and to nurses considering a change of practice into ambulatory surgery.

CHAPTER 1

OVERVIEW OF AMBULATORY SURGERY

CHAPTER OBJECTIVE

Upon completion of this chapter, the reader will be able to discuss how changes in the health care delivery system in the past century have influenced the utilization of ambulatory surgery.

LEARNING OBJECTIVES

After studying the material in this chapter, the reader will be able to

1. differentiate between types of ambulatory surgery facilities.
2. list reasons for consumer acceptance of ambulatory surgery.
3. identify trends expected to influence ambulatory surgery in the future.
4. recognize the evolving role of nursing in ambulatory surgery.

INTRODUCTION

Advances in surgical technology as well as the development of shorter acting anesthetics and ancillary drugs have facilitated the performance of more complex procedures in ambulatory surgical settings. Concomitantly, the impact of managed care, pressure from third-party payers, and patient preferences have caused a rapid expansion in the number of ambulatory surgical procedures performed in the past 15 to 20 years. In 2008 there were more than 5,000 ambulatory surgery centers (ASCs) in the United States that provided more than 22 million procedures (Ambulatory Surgery Center Associations [ASC], n.d.-b).

EVOLUTION OF AMBULATORY CARE

Now widely accepted, even mandated by third-party payers for certain procedures, the concept of ambulatory surgery was slow to gain appreciation and acceptance.

As early as 1910, when 21 days of bed rest was routinely prescribed convalescence after inguinal herniorrhaphy, Drs. Emil Ries of Chicago and Herman Boldt of New York, both gynecologic surgeons, were advocating early ambulation following laparotomy and pelvic surgery. Dr. Ries noted that patients, who were allowed out of bed in 24 to 48 hours and were discharged in less than a week did not have the muscular weakness and listlessness characteristic of longer postoperative confinement. Nevertheless, this premise failed to gain support in the surgical community.

In February 1918, the first outpatient general anesthesia in the United States was successfully administered by Ralph Waters, an anesthesiologist, at the Down-Town Anesthesia Clinic he established in an office building in Sioux City, Iowa. Local surgeons performed relatively minor procedures there, such as setting fractures, draining abscesses, and performing dental surgery. In a paper he presented later that year at a medical meeting in Indianapolis, Waters commented that costs for outpatient surgery were considerably less than costs for similar procedures done in a hospital.

Still, the concept of ambulatory, or outpatient surgery, was largely ignored for several decades.

By the 1950s, socialized health care in the United Kingdom was causing extraordinary delays of up to 2 years for elective surgery. This situation led some surgeons to recognize that ambulatory surgery, which was being successfully used for children, could be equally applicable to many adult procedures. As a result, a pivotal study by J.A. Stallworthy, the well known Oxford gynecologist, advocating decreasing postoperative hospitalization was published in *The Lancet* in 1960 (Schirmer & Rattner, 1998). It was titled "Hotels or Hospitals."

In the United States, ambulatory surgery gained impetus in the 1960s and hospital-based or affiliated facilities began to be established. One of the keys to this growth was the acceptance of the idea that anesthesia could be safely administered in an ambulatory setting. Anesthesiologists David Cohen and John Dillon championed the premise that judicious patient assessment and selection, combined with safe anesthetic and surgical techniques, led to successful ambulatory surgical procedures. They were instrumental in the opening of one of the earliest, widely publicized units at the Center for Health Services at the University of California at Los Angeles (UCLA) in 1962.

By 1966, *The Journal of the American Medical Association* (*JAMA*) stated that it was possible to conduct a program of anesthesia for outpatient surgery without compromising patient safety. In 1968, a United States National Advisory Commission on Health Facilities report advocated experiments to help decrease health care costs (Federated Ambulatory Surgery Association [FASA], 1998).

In 1970, the first successful freestanding ASC was opened in Phoenix, Arizona. The Surgicenter, founded by anesthesiologists Wallace Reed and John Ford in conjunction with a nurse, Sharon Schafer (DeFazio-Quinn, 1997), served as a model for future outpatient surgery centers. The success, acceptance, and promotion of the Surgicenter were key factors in the rapid expansion of ambulatory surgical facilities during the decade (Schirmer & Rattner, 1998). Later that year, a second ASC opened, and more than 5,700 surgeries were performed at these two centers during the year.

The American Medical Association (AMA) passed a resolution in 1971 that endorsed the concept of outpatient surgery under general and local anesthesia for selected procedures and patients. In 1973, the American Society of Anesthesiologists (ASA) published *Guidelines for Ambulatory Surgery Facilities.*

In 1972 the Department of Health, Education, and Welfare received a mandate from Congress to do a feasibility study for reimbursing freestanding ambulatory surgery facilities. Done by the Orkland Corporation, the study confirmed that surgery could be accomplished safely and less expensively in freestanding facilities on an outpatient basis. By 1974 a contract was signed for a Medicare demonstration project with six surgery centers. Sixty-seven surgery centers were operating in the United States by 1976 (FASA, 1998).

Major medical and surgical advances were made during the decades since 1950, and as technology proliferated, so too did health care costs. Federally funded Medicare and Medicaid programs added more monetary stimulation for expansion of health care services until, in the 1970s, concerns about escalating costs started to be addressed. The recognition that safe health care had to be delivered more economically spurred the growth of ambulatory care programs through the 1980s and into the current decade.

More than 900 ASCs opened during the decade of the 1980s, bringing the total number to 1,200.

The number of ASCs has increased commensurately with the expansion of Medicare procedures approved for an ASC setting. In 1982, the federal government began approving Medicare payment for patients having surgery in ASCs. At that time there were approximately 200 covered procedures; currently there are more than 2,500 Medicare-approved procedures. Medicare patients receive approximately 30% of care provided in ASCs (ASC, n.d.-a).

Insurance companies have tried to influence patients to choose ambulatory surgery by covering only a portion of the surgical fee for an inpatient procedure but providing full coverage for the same procedure if performed as an outpatient. In some cases insurers completely deny coverage for certain procedures if they are not performed on an ambulatory basis (Schirmer & Rattner, 1998). Private payers, especially managed care plans, continue to drive ASC expansion because of the efficiencies and savings realized.

Based on 2007 Medicare data, the most commonly performed procedures in the Medicare population include ophthalmologic surgery (31%), gastroenterology (35%), orthopedic surgery (7%), and general surgery (4%). For nonMedicare eligible populations, 3% of procedures are gynecological, 3% are plastic surgery, 8% are ear/nose/throat, and 5% are general surgery. Forty two percent of ASCs specialize in a particular type of surgery, with 58% providing multiple types of procedures (ASC, n.d.-b).

A 2006 survey of 250 freestanding ASCs across the country – representing more than one million cases – found that gastroenterology and orthopedic procedures accounted for 25% and 18% respectively of all cases performed. These, together with ophthalmology, pain management, and otolaryngology comprised nearly 80% of the total case volume. Associated revenues in each category per case were: orthopedics $2,136; GI $749; ophthalmology $1,145; pain management $830; and ENT $1536 (Informed Health Choices, 2006).

TYPES OF AMBULATORY SURGICAL FACILITIES

Ambulatory surgical facilities are usually divided into three categories: hospital-based, hospital-affiliated or satellite, and freestanding. Considering the amount of surgery performed in physician office facilities, it would seem reasonable to consider office-based ambulatory surgery as a fourth category. According to The Federation of State Medical Boards (2002), in the United States, more operations are done as outpatient (65%) than as inpatient (35%). It is estimated that 15% to 20% of all outpatient operations are being done as office-based surgeries.

The earliest ambulatory surgeries were performed in hospital-based facilities. Scheduling and administration were commingled with inpatient surgery. Late running inpatient schedules or emergencies impacted and usually took precedence over outpatient procedures, leading to frustration for staff, patients, and surgeons. However, the hospital setting provided a major advantage because resources such as equipment, central bill processing, and pharmacy services could be utilized as needed.

An advantage for the patient in a hospital-based facility is the availability of overnight admission should that become advisable. For this reason, surgical procedures of greater magnitude can be performed in this setting. These advantages also apply to a hospital-affiliated unit with autonomous perioperative and operative areas and dedicated staff, a setup which is more client-friendly and cost-effective.

On the other hand, freestanding ASCs provide ease of parking, a less-complicated campus to maneuver, less opportunity for delays in the surgical schedule and a staff that has a single focus toward ambulatory procedures. Freestanding surgery centers are versatile in the scope of services and convenience provided to patients. According to a study by the U.S. Department of Health and Human Services Office of the Inspector General OIG, Medicare patients prefer ASCs to hospitals for outpatient surgical and diagnostic procedures. Among reasons for this preference was less waiting time, less crowded and more comfortable environments, lower costs, less paperwork, and a more convenient location and parking (ASC, n.d.-c). Effective May 18, 2009, Medicare defines an ASC as "any distinct entity that operates exclusively for the purpose of providing surgical services to patients not requiring hospitalization and in which the expected duration of services would not exceed 24 hours following an admission" (CMS, 2009, p. 31).

Recovery Care Centers

Recovery care centers (RCCs) provide postsurgical care for a defined length of time based on individual state regulations. First offered in 1984 in a single ambulatory surgical facility in Coeur D'Alene, Idaho, by 1996 extended postsurgical recovery was being offered in 9.6% of freestanding ASCs. Some states allow patients to remain in the facility for up to 23 hours after outpatient surgery, 0.05% offered 72-hour recovery. Prior to RCCs, complex surgical procedures, in which it was possible that the patient might require extended postoperative care, could not be done in ASCs (FASA, n.d.).

Recognizing that patients may need extended observation and intervention because of potential bleeding, impaired circulation of an extremity, or pain management, the American Society of PeriAnesthesia Nurses (ASPAN) developed standards of practice for nursing care for what is referred to as phase III recovery (Clifford, Mamaril, & Sullivan, 2005). RCCs allow more types of surgery, such as laminectomies, laparoscopic assisted vaginal hysterectomies, and mastectomies to be done in freestanding centers. FASA noted in correspondence to the administrator of the Centers for Medicare and Medicaid Services (CMS) that for two decades RCCs affiliated with ASCs have facilitated the use of technological advances to safely perform many types of surgeries for patients of all age-groups (FASA, 2007). Although, some states regulations have prohibited facilities from keeping patients overnight, postsurgical recovery care represents a fast growing trend (FASA, n.d.). Medicare does not yet reimburse for recovery care services.

An alternative to providing recovery care in RCCs is the provision for patients to stay in a nearby hotel overnight and receive care from a home health nurse. In a study done on patients undergoing laparoscopic Nissen fundoplication, the home health nurse stayed with the patient 1 to 3 hours after transfer to the hotel and then made a second visit in late evening. The surgeon also visited the patient, and a family member or friend stayed with the patient overnight. No complications occurred, and patient satisfaction was high (Cohn, Klinger, & Hinder, 1997). A variety of extended recovery settings may be categorized as Phase III settings (Clifford, Mamaril, & Sullivan, 2005).

COST CONTAINMENT

In the United States, ambulatory surgery was born of the need for cost containment. Health care costs continue to outpace inflation, which makes options to costly hospitalization imperative. Cost outcomes for ambulatory surgery are typically assessed by comparing the inpatient versus outpatient costs of a particular procedure. To establish the total societal cost, the amount of time away from normal daily activity plus the dollar value of the time expended by nonprofessional caregivers must be considered.

ASCs have been able to provide quality care more economically than hospitals because they have low overhead costs and they focus on one area: treating ambulatory patients efficiently. On average, procedures performed in an ASC cost 47% less than the same procedure performed in a hospital (ASC, n.d.-c). Patients usually pay less coinsurance in an ASC.

For example, a Medicare beneficiary typically would pay $496 coinsurance for a cataract extraction in a hospital, but the copayment in an ASC would be $195. For a colonoscopy, a Medicare beneficiary typically pays a $186 copayment in a hospital, but $89 in an ASC (MedPAC, 2004). An earlier study done by Blue Cross and Blue Shield found that facility fees for removal of tonsils cost an average of $464 in an ASC, compared with $998 if performed in a hospital (ASC, n.d.-c).

Similarly, cataract surgery costs averaged $835 in an ASC, compared with $2,012 in a hospital, and an inguinal herniorrhaphy done in an ASC cost $601 versus $1,271 as an inpatient (ASC, n.d.-c). Cost containment will continue to be a challenge and facilities must be prepared to deal with third party and Medicare payment systems.

The CMS projects hospital outpatient services costs to be more than $32 billion for 2007. The Medicare Modernization Act required implementation of a modernized payment system for ASCs by 2008. This legislation should allow every surgical procedure that can be safely performed in an ASC to be listed in the ASC payment system (CMS, 2006).

ACCREDITATION

Increasingly, ambulatory surgical facilities are seeking accreditation, motivated by economics and ethics. Accreditation strengthens third-party reimbursement negotiations; health care payers expect providers to qualitatively document that patients receive the care and service for which they contracted. The scrutiny of consumer advocates and special interest groups associated with the legal and insurance industries provide an additional incentive.

The most stringent accreditation guidelines for ambulatory surgery facilities are those of the federal government for Medicare reimbursement (Schirmer & Rattner, 1998). Currently, 43 states require state ASC licensure as well.

Accrediting agencies, such as The Joint Commission and the Accreditation Association for Ambulatory Health Care (AAAHC) set benchmark standards of care. In the legal system, these standards are admitted as evidence to determine the legal standard of care that is relied on as authoritative by physicians and others providing ambulatory surgical care. Joint Commission and AAAHC standards are comprehensive and authoritative and are given the same evidentiary weight in litigation (Ireland, 1997).

In the past several years, Joint Commission standards have become less prescriptive and more process oriented. Requirements are now more functionally oriented for system-wide performance and involve all health care practitioners on staff. The standards address 12 major areas.

- Patient rights
- Organization ethics
- Assessment of patients
- Care of patients
- Education of patients and family
- Continuum of care
- Improvement of organizational performance
- Leadership
- Management of environmental care
- Management of human resources
- Management of information
- Surveillance, prevention, and control of infection

The AAAHC's program of standards and procedures for credentials verification organizations is intended to provide health care organizations with resources for verifying the professional credentials and experience of physicians and other licensed independent health care practitioners providing services on their medical staffs. AAAHC was also the first accrediting body to develop laser technology standards and standards for pediatric anesthesia and surgery (AAAHC, 1998).

Another accrediting organization is the American Association for Accreditation of Ambulatory Surgery Facilities, Inc. (AAAASF). Based on inquiries by other surgical specialties, the AAAASF was formed in 1992 to accredit other single specialty and multi-specialty surgery facilities owned and/or operated by surgeons of other specialties who are certified by a surgical specialty board of the American Board of Medical Specialists (ABMS). The rigid requirements are the same for each specialty, and, in addition to certification as a surgeon specialist, each surgeon at the facility must hold unrestricted hospital privileges in his or her local community in the specialty in which he or she is practicing and participate in a peer review program. A quality assessment and quality improvement program must be maintained, and all personnel must meet facility standards of the accredited program (AAAASF, 2006).

As office-based surgery became an increasingly significant part of the practice, the American Society of Plastic and Reconstructive Surgeons realized the importance of ensuring high standards, not only for physicians through board certification, but for office-based ambulatory surgical facilities in which 70% to 80% of plastic surgeons practiced. Consequently, in 1980, the society established the American Association for Accreditation of Ambulatory Plastic Surgery Facilities (AAAAPSF) to design and operate a single specialty accreditation program for outpatient plastic surgery centers (AAAASF, 1998).

Ambulatory care facilities are also accredited by class, based on three-tiered classifications of anesthesia administered. Class A accreditation requires that all surgical procedures performed in the facility be done under local or topical anesthesia. For Class AB, the use of intravenous or parenteral sedation, regional anesthesia, analgesics, or dissociative drugs is added, but without the use of endotracheal or laryngeal mask intubation or the use of inhalation general anesthesia. Class ABC includes the stipulations of the previous two classes and also the use of endotracheal or laryngeal mask intubation or inhalation anesthesia administered by an anesthesiologist or certified registered nurse anesthetist (CRNA). These definitive criteria are very important to the safety and well-being of the patient, as discussed in following chapters.

California was the first state to require surgical facilities that perform procedures using general anesthesia or agents that may "compromise the patient's life-protective reflexes" to be accredited, Medicare certified, or licensed as a surgery center by the state's Department of Health Services. Considered model legislation when introduced in 1996, similar laws and regulations were adopted soon after by Florida, Georgia, New Jersey, Pennsylvania, and Texas (AAAASF, 2006).

Although the Comprehensive Accreditation Manual for Ambulatory Care applies to all types of ambulatory facilities, The Joint Commission developed quality standards expressly for accreditation of office-based surgery practices that became effective January 1, 2001 (JCAHO, 2000a). Similarly, California, Florida, Pennsylvania, Rhode Island, Texas, and New Jersey drafted legislation dealing with office-based surgery. Prompted by media coverage of adverse events in office-based surgical facilities, other states began implementing regulatory requirements through their Departments of Health or state Boards of Medicine (Aker, 2001).

In October 2006, Oregon became the 22nd state to regulate office-based surgery. One of the stipulations is that the licensed practitioner who performs a procedure must determine if the patient is ready to be discharged safely from the office. Similarly, the Illinois Department of Public Health has issued a proposal that would require a qualified physician to be present in the ASC until all patients are medically discharged (Percy, 2007).

In July 2007, the state of New York passed a law requiring all doctors performing office-based surgery that necessitates moderate to deep sedation or anesthesia to have their office reviewed and accredited by July 2009 or face penalties from the state medical board. Additionally, as of January 2008 all adverse events must be reported to the state Department of Health (AAAHC, 2006).

NURSING PERSPECTIVES

The scope of practice for ambulatory surgical nurses presents considerable challenges. Unlike the hospital setting where patient populations and disease entities are stratified for specialized care, an ASC requires the nurse be prepared to skillfully care for diverse age-groups, varying levels of patient wellness, and multi specialty procedures.

In the fast-paced, cost-conscious ambulatory surgery environment, nurses function in all phases of perioperative patient care, from admission to discharge. Core and critical nursing intervention skills are necessary to assess, plan, implement, and evaluate an individualized care plan for each patient. Ambulatory care nursing requires a high level of autonomy, critical thinking, and leadership skills (American Academy of Ambulatory Care Nursing [AAACN], n.d.).

High-quality patient care consistent with established standards of practice must be delivered, but public relations, business, and time-management issues must also be addressed by the ASC nurse. In an ambulatory surgical setting, teamwork is essential and collaboration with other disciplines is important. The successful ASC depends on collaborative relationships and mutual respect among all members of the health care team (Brockway, 1997). Safe high-quality patient care depends to a great degree on a clinical team's ability to communicate effectively (The Joint Commission, 2006b).

As nurse-patient contact time decreases, the nurse's role as a teacher must be emphasized to ensure that patients and caregivers are well informed and adequately prepared to deal with the added responsibility they assume after discharge. Nurses practicing in ambulatory surgical care settings are patient advocates committed to the safety and comfort of patients of all age-groups (Kolcaba & Wilson, 2002). As technology escalates and the complexity of procedures performed in the ASC grows the nurse's continuing educational commitment becomes essential to maintaining competency. Joint Commission Standard HR 4.2 points out that ongoing in-service and other education and training maintain and improve staff competency.

Credentialing is the process of setting performance standards and then awarding the right to care for patients on the basis of those standards. Certification of individual ambulatory health care workers depends on state law, community standards of practice, and the organizational structure of the facility. Generally, certification requirements for ASC medical staff are the same as those required by hospitals for similar positions.

Employed health care providers must also meet standards and competencies. In 2006, the Association of periOperative Registered Nurses (AORN) launched a legislative initiative to have individual states pass a Registered Nurse Circulator bill, which would require circulators in ASC operating rooms to be registered nurses (AAAHC, 2006).

For Joint Commission accreditation, competency verification became mandatory in 1993. In a health care organization, each individual must be competent in the knowledge and skills required to perform his or her responsibilities; in effective use of all equipment used in his or her activities; and in cardiopulmonary resuscitation (CPR) and other lifesaving interventions. Individuals must also demonstrate competency in preventing contamination and transfer of infection.

Standards for specialized areas of practice are typically defined by professional organizations. For the ambulatory surgery and perianesthesia nurse, the AORN, the ASPAN, the American Nurses Association (ANA), and the American Academy of Ambulatory Care Nursing all provide guidance. For example, ASPAN provides national nursing standards of practice, and AORN publishes *Recommended Practices on Managing the Patient Receiving Conscious Sedation/Analgesia*. Some state nurse practice acts specifically address ambulatory nursing.

The American Board of Perianesthesia Nursing Certification, Inc. (ABPANC) was established by ASPAN in 1985 to administer certification programs for qualified registered nurses. Its mission is "assuring a certification process, for perianesthesia nurses, which validates knowledge gained through professional education and experience, ultimately promoting quality patient care." The organization is committed to evidence-based practice.

ABPANC offers two certification programs: the certified postanesthesia nurse (CPAN) and the certified ambulatory perianesthesia nurse (CAPA) designations (ABPANC, n.d.).

SUMMARY

In this country 70% of all surgeries are outpatient procedures and one of every five of them are done in an ASC. As technical innovations continue to advance, more and more surgical procedures will be suitable for ASC settings. The aggressive use of minimally invasive surgical techniques is expected to allow a continued shift to outpatient facilities. Cardiac surgery, one of the most costly of inpatient procedures, is already increasing on an outpatient basis. Expansion of microsurgery is expected, and improved imaging techniques will offer new venues. For example, innovations in magnetic resonance imaging may increase early surgical interventions in cancer care. As the number of older adults continues to increase, so too will the number of ambulatory endoscopic, ophthalmic, and arthroscopic procedures.

As changes in the types of and settings for ambulatory surgery take place, nurses practicing in ambulatory surgical settings will be challenged to grow and adapt while preserving the art of caring and the therapeutic science of nursing (Clifford, Mamaril, & Sullivan, 2005).

EXAM QUESTIONS

CHAPTER 1

Questions 1-9

Note: Choose the option that BEST answers each question.

1. A key factor in the growth of ambulatory surgery was the recognition that
   a. general anesthesia could be safely administered to outpatients.
   b. profits would decrease proportionately.
   c. insurance companies would not negotiate.
   d. less equipment would be required.

2. In the United States, the Surgicenter in Phoenix, Arizona, is generally recognized as being the first successful
   a. hospital-based ambulatory surgery facility.
   b. hospital-affiliated ambulatory surgery facility.
   c. freestanding ambulatory surgery center.
   d. government-approved ambulatory surgery center.

3. The U.S. federal government began approving Medicare payment for surgery performed in ambulatory surgical centers in
   a. 1962.
   b. 1975.
   c. 1982.
   d. 1985.

4. The most frequently performed procedures in ambulatory facilities have been
   a. gynecologic.
   b. ophthalmologic.
   c. neurologic.
   d. cosmetic.

5. In the United States, ambulatory surgery expanded because of the need for
   a. fewer hospital beds.
   b. cost containment.
   c. fewer nurses.
   d. less equipment.

6. Medicare does not reimburse for
   a. recovery care services.
   b. freestanding surgical care services.
   c. diagnostic surgical procedures.
   d. emergency surgical procedures.

7. Ambulatory surgical centers (ASCs) have been able to provide quality care more economically than hospitals because they
   a. charge higher copayments.
   b. charge insurers higher rates.
   c. have fewer licensed staff.
   d. have lower overhead costs.

8. As nurse-patient contact time decreases, which topic should be emphasized?
   a. Discharge criteria
   b. Ancillary staff
   c. Patient teaching
   d. Premedication

9. As the number of older adults increases, the number of which type of procedure is expected to increase?

   a. Dental
   b. Gynecologic
   c. Endoscopic
   d. Fluoroscopic

pg 8

CHAPTER 2

PATIENT SELECTION AND EVALUATION

CHAPTER OBJECTIVE

Upon completion of this chapter, the reader will be able to describe the selection of and preoperative assessment for the ambulatory surgical patient.

LEARNING OBJECTIVES

After studying this chapter, the reader will be able to

1. identify essential components of preoperative patient assessments and procedures.
2. recognize the psychological and emotional concerns of patients.
3. assess patient and caregiver learning needs.

INTRODUCTION

Thorough and comprehensive preoperative evaluation of the prospective ambulatory surgical patient is essential for perioperative management and positive outcomes. Similarly, the importance of teaching patients before surgery about what may be expected after surgery should not be overlooked. Preoperative instruction may reduce anxiety and aid in coping, which results in enhanced postoperative recovery (Pasero & Beiden, 2006). Ambulatory surgery patients should be assessed as a hospitalized patient would be, relative to the surgical procedure and patient's physical condition.

THE SELECTION PROCESS

When ambulatory surgery became popular, eligible patients were limited to those qualifying as class P1 and P2 according to the American Society of Anesthesiologists (ASA) physical status classification (see Table 2-1). Increasingly, medically stable class P3 patients became recognized as suitable for ambulatory surgery. In selected cases, largely due to third-party payer reimbursement policies, physically less stable patients may also be candidates for outpatient procedures. Patient and procedure selection begins in the surgeon's office. The surgeon, anesthesiologist, and sometimes other physician consultants evaluate the patient's physical consition and tolerance for the procedure and the anesthetic (Burden, 2000).

Types of Surgery

As ambulatory surgery evolves, complications and unplanned hospital admissions have been found to correlate with the type and duration of surgery as well as the physical status or age of the patient. The type of procedure that may be performed in ambulatory surgery depends more on postoperative patient requirements for specialized care and pain management along with the possibility of complications than on intraoperative factors (White & Durieux, 2005). The following general list includes conditions that may cause a surgical procedure to be considered unsuitable on an ambulatory basis:

TABLE 2-1: ASA PHYSICAL STATUS CLASSIFICATION SYSTEM

P1 — A normal healthy patient

P2 — A patient with mild systemic disease

P3 — A patient with severe systemic disease

P4 — A patient with severe systemic disease that is a constant threat to life

P5 — A moribund patient who is not expected to survive without the operation

P6 — A declared brain-dead patient whose organs are being removed for donor purposes

The above six levels are consistent with the American Society of Anesthesiologists ranking of patient physical status.

Note. Excerpted from *1998 Relative Value Guide of the American Society of Anesthesiologists*. A copy of the full text can be obtained from ASA, 520 N. Northwest Highway, Park Ridge, Illinois 60068-2573. Reprinted with permission.

- Involvement of a part of an organ system that causes incapacity in the entire system from which the patient must recover. For example, intra-articular knee surgery on only one leg is acceptable, whereas resection of even a short segment of bowel causes generalized ileus and is unacceptable.
- Resulting external or internal fluid shift that requires prolonged observation and intravenous (IV) replacement postoperatively. An example is massive liposuction.
- Interference with and requirement for adjustment of the medical treatment of a concurrent unstable illness.
- Prevention of the patient from oral intake, necessitating IV therapy to maintain fluid balance.
- Resulting pain sufficient to warrant IV, intramuscular (IM), epidural, or intrathecal drug administration in the extended recovery period.
- Resulting need for drug administration regularly by the parenteral route, as with IV antibiotics for infection or subcutaneous heparin as a prophylaxis against thrombosis (Chung & Lam, 1997).
- Requirement for invasive monitoring.

Surgical procedures that involve major blood loss or require general anesthesia for longer than 4 hours may also be inappropriate. There is considerable controversy concerning tonsillectomies and adenoidectomies (T & A) performed in an outpatient setting because 3% of these patients experience postoperative bleeding, some of which require transfusion and reoperation.

In very young children, post-tonsillectomy breathing problems and nausea and vomiting leading to dehydration are additional concerns. After T & A, patients also may be prone to laryngospasm, so adedquate postoperative monitoring is essential. (Drain, 2009). Surgical location must be decided on a case-by-case basis after careful evaluation. Decisions are influenced by the type of ambulatory facility, the skill and resources of those caring for the patient, postoperative resources, and community standards.

Patient Selection

Whether a patient is appropriate for ambulatory surgery is a clinical decision made by the physicians involved in care. In many facilities the medical oversight committee may develop a standard, guideline or policy about patient appropriateness based on the particular ambulatory setting.

Adult patients typically considered appropriate for ambulatory surgery include healthy patients without systemic disease and those with stable chronic conditions such as well-controlled diabetes or stable cardiac or pulmonary disease.

Some of the conditions that may deem a person as inappropriate for ambulatory surgery include:

- Patients with unstable chronic diseases such as:
  - poorly controlled insulin-dependent diabetics
  - congestive heart failure or unstable angina
  - acute exacerbations of chronic lung disease

- Morbidly obese patients with symptomatic respiratory or cardiovascular problems
- Patients with a compromised airway
- Patients receiving centrally active drug therapy, such as monoamine oxidase (MAO) inhibitors
- Active cocaine abusers (because of increased risk of intraoperative cardiovascular complications)
- Patients with mediastinal masses
- ASA class P3 and P4 patients who require complex or extended monitoring or postoperative treatment
- Patients with an anticipated need for complex postoperative pain management
- Patients with significant fever, nasal congestion, cough, or wheezing indicating a recent upper respiratory infection (URI).
- Developmentally challenged patients who are not able to follow postoperative instructions and who are without continued responsible adult care at home or in an aftercare facility.
- Patients with obstructive sleep apnea (OSA), whose suitability remains controversial (Joshi, 2006).

Pediatric patients considered unsuitable for ambulatory surgery include:

- Formerly premature infants of less than 46 weeks' postconception age (gestational age plus postnatal age) because of increased risk of postoperative apnea
- Very young children with respiratory disease or dysfunction such as:
  - severe bronchopulmonary dysplasia
  - apneic episodes
  - recurrent bronchospasm
- Infants with cardiovascular disease such as:
  - congestive heart failure
  - hemodynamically significant congenital heart anomalies
- Children with fever, cough, sore throat, coryza, or other signs of recent onset or worsening URI
- Children who are siblings of sudden infant death syndrome (SIDS) victims

Physiologic status is more of a determining factor of an appropriate candidate for ambulatory surgery than is chronological age. With the exception of infants who were born prematurely, where experts believe acceptable postconception age for outpatient surgery varies from 44 to 60 weeks, extremes of age are no longer considered a contraindication to ambulatory surgery if the patient is healthy.

Eligibility for ambulatory surgery must be decided on a case-by-case basis. ASA class P3 patients may be suitable for outpatient procedures if the concurrent systemic disease is well controlled. Morbidly obese patients present potential airway maintenance problems and typically have numerous medical concerns, including sleep apnea. However, for short procedures with cautious anesthetic management, ambulatory surgery may be acceptable.

Appropriateness of patients with a personal or family history of malignant hyperthermia (MH) is another topic of controveresy. Any patient may present with an MH response unexpectedly after anesthesia has begun. With the availability of short-acting IV agents that do not trigger MH, it may be possible to safely anesthetize patients with a known genetic predisposition to this disease in ambulatory settings for short surgical procedures. Selection of the patient and procedure for ambulatory surgery in large part depends on the surgical facility, quality of postoperative care, and community standards of practice. Patients susceptible to MH should be observed postoperatively for a minimum of 4 hours before discharge (White & Recart-Friere, 2005).

As the number of overweight individuals increases, so too does the incidence of OSA, which develops in children as well as adults. OSA may impact every phase of the perioperative experience, and increased morbidity and mortality have been associated with management preparation. It is estimated that 80% of cases of OSA are undiagnosed

(Joshi, 2006). Consequently, during the preoperative evaluation the nurse should be particularly alert for signs and patient comments suggesting OSA, including: history of loud snoring; brief apneic arousals during sleep; fatigue; chronic sleepiness despite adequate "sleep" time; tendency to fall asleep easily when watching television, reading, riding, or driving; and hypertension (Moos & Cuddeford, 2006).

It should also be noted that increased neck girth increases the likelihood of OSA. Whether or not the patient has ever had a sleep study, along with results should be noted on the chart. Those who have had corrective airway surgery should be assumed to be at risk unless sleep studies and symptoms have normalized (Joshi, 2006). Any patient with suspected or diagnosed OSA should have a thorough preoperative anesthesia evaluation before the day of surgery.

Patients who use continuous positive airway pressure (CPAP) therapy should be asked to bring their device on the day of surgery for possible postoperative use. If this is not permitted by the ASC, the nurse should document the precise settings currently used by the patient, including the possible use of supplemental oxygen. Facility-approved CPAP equipments with the appropriate settings must be available at the time of surgery (Moos & Cuddeford, 2006)

PREOPERATIVE PATIENT ASSESSMENT

Adequate preoperative assessment of the prospective ambulatory surgical patient is essential for optimal perioperative management and outcome. By identifying existing or potential areas of concern, the goal of having the patient in the best possible health consistent with his or her physical status at the time of surgery may be achieved. In addition to gathering the necessary information, the nurse's role focuses on preparing the patient physically and emotionally.

Assessment and evaluation may be accomplished by a patient visit to the facility prior to the day of surgery, an office visit, a telephone interview, a written questionnaire, a computer-aided survey (e.g., Health Quiz) completed by the patient, or surgical and anesthetic assessment done the morning of surgery. The last method usually has the highest cancellation rate (White & Recart-Friere, 2005).

Assessment is best performed sufficiently in advance of the scheduled surgery to allow time for investigation of areas of concern, obtaining previous medical records and consultations if needed. The greatest advantage of a facility visit is that it allows adequate time for a thorough preoperative evaluation to be performed and consultations to be obtained as indicated (Hwang, Bill, & Edlich, 1998). However, this visit may be inconvenient for the patient, so telephone interviews are frequently used in ambulatory facilities. It is important for the telephone interview to be conducted at least 1 to 2 days in advance of the scheduled surgery, by a registered nurse who can evaluate the patient for appropriateness for ambulatory surgery and identify the need for any tests that could not be performed the day of surgery. The perioperative nurse should review results of preprocedure diagnostic tests and notify the surgeon of any questionable abnormalities. Ambulatory surgery patients should be assessed as a hospitalized patient would be, relative to the surgical procedure and patient's physical condition. The best disease screening procedures continue to be a carefully performed physical examination along with a detailed history. Based on the results, laboratory testing may then be ordered. A battery of unnecessary tests is not cost effective and may increase patient anxiety.

Ambulatory facilities may have protocols for minimum assessment information and laboratory values required preoperatively. These parameters may include vital signs; hemoglobin and hematocrit; oxygen saturation; chest x-ray; electrocardiogram (ECG); and medication history, including substance abuse. For a geriatric patient, blood urea nitrogen (BUN) may be added. Obtaining a potassium level is advisable for patients on diuretics because hypokalemia may cause dangerous dysrhythmias, especially if hypoxemia develops during surgery or in the postanesthesia care unit (PACU).

Several standard-setting organizations, such as the American College of Physicians (ACP), the American College of Surgeons (ACS), and the ASA have developed recommendations for preoperative patient evaluation. According to the ASA, appropriate indications for ordering tests include the identification of specific clinical indicators or risk factors such as age, preexisting disease, or magnitude of the surgical procedure.

A chest x-ray and ECG may be necessary only if warranted by the patient's history or age. Additionally, previous tests showing normal results may be acceptable. A chest x-ray within 1 year, ECG within 6 months, or blood tests done within 6 weeks prior to surgery may be satisfactory if there has been no intervening clinical event. The Joint Commission stipulates (PC 13.20) that a history and physical must have been done no more than 30 days prior to the day of surgery. Medicare and state licensing regulations may involve additional requirements. In healthy male outpatients scheduled for procedures such as arthroscopy or herniorrhaphy, laboratory tests may not be needed; however, a hemoglobin or hematocrit test may be advisable for females (White & Recart-Friere, 2005).

Females of childbearing age should be asked about the possibility of pregnancy, and their last menstrual period should be documented. If there is any question of pregnancy, some facilities require testing prior to surgery.

For children, birth history and developmental stage may be included. Height and weight in kilograms should be documented. Head circumference of infants is another facet that may be part of the preoperative assessment in some institutions. Healthy children more than 12 months old, who are scheduled for surgery that does not have a significant potential for blood loss, do not require any blood tests unless clinically indicated (Hwang et al., 1998). However, for children undergoing chemotherapy, a hemoglobin or hematocrit test is advisable (White & Recart-Friere, 2005).

African American children younger than age 15 should be tested for sickle cell anemia. Because this disease is usually diagnosed in early childhood, preoperative testing may not be necessary for the patient age 15 and older. If positive for sickle cell anemia, the patient should be free from infection, hydrated, and hemodynamically stable before surgery. Any patient in acute crisis is unsuitable for ambulatory surgery (Litwack, 1997).

The nurse's assessment should consider the patient's emotional status, cognitive ability, and social or cultural influences. The alert perioperative nurse will add and document physical or mental impairments or disabilities; communication limitations; mobility limitations; and prostheses used, including hearing aids and contact lenses. If a patient has a pacemaker, the type should be documented on the patient's chart. For a patient with an implantable cardiac defibrillator (ICD), there should be an external defibrillator readily available during surgery and recovery. The ASA recommends a preoperative evaluation of any device in a patient having elective surgery; ideally, the evaluation is repeated after the procedure (Rozner, 2006).

Skillful interviewing techniques and the ability to discern what the patient may have neglected to mention may make the difference between a safe and uneventful ambulatory surgical experience and an emergency situation. This is especially true with elderly patients who may not want to admit that they do not understand, do not hear well, or have forgotten certain information. How the question is phrased is often the key to patient response.

Specific questions asked in a pleasant, nonthreatening, and unhurried manner are most effective.

Seemingly conversational questions may provide valuable insights. For example, in talking with patients with known systemic diseases, questions about sports and hobbies (e.g., gardening), may provide a gauge of exercise tolerance, functional physiologic reserve, and stress tolerance. The presence of stairs in the home or estimates of housework performed may provide similar insight. For smokers, a discussion of morning routine and smoking habits facilitates an estimation of the degree of chronic respiratory compromise and may also lead to discovery of cessation adjuncts the patient is using but neglected to mention.

Questions about allergies or side effects to medications require more direct approach. Patients tend to describe nausea and other gastrointestinal upsets secondary to medications as allergies rather than side effects. Side effects involve unpleasant or adverse reactions. Allergic reactions are characterized by hives, pruritus, skin wheals, edema, wheezing, bronchospasms, hypotension, or circulatory collapse (Kost, 2004).

Latex sensitivity should be specifically addressed. If the patient is not aware of latex sensitivity, he or she should be asked about redness, itching, or swelling after wearing rubber gloves; dental, vaginal, or rectal examinations; or blowing up balloons. A positive response warrants further investigation, and the surgeon and anesthesia provider should be notified. Additionally, the ambulatory surgery staff should be prepared to establish a latex-safe environment. A history of developing a rash after touching poinsettia plants or reactions to tropical fruits such as avocados, bananas, or kiwi may indicate possible latex sensitivity. Any child with a confirmed allergy to bananas should be considered to be allergic to latex (American Association of Nurse Anesthetists [AANA], 2001). Allergies to chestnuts, tomatoes, and potatoes have also been associated with the risk of latex sensitivity (Noble, 2005)

Similarly, allergy to seafood is a contraindication to the use of iodine compounds such as contrast agents for radiologic procedures, protamine sulfate, and betadine preparations. Allergy to eggs may be a contraindication to the use of propofol (Diprivan) for sedation or anesthesia (Dunn, 1998).

Patients are often unclear about previous procedures; they may believe they had general anesthesia, when in fact they slept after sedation and regional anesthesia. The type of procedure and description of events are significant indications of what questions should follow. However, prolonged or incapacitating nausea and vomiting is not usually forgotten. Patients should be questioned about recovery from previous anesthetics and procedures so that precautions may be taken to avoid repetition of any adverse effects. Broad generalizations, such as an allergy to "penicillin" or "sleeping pills," must be defined.

Similarly, the patient should be specifically asked about a personal or family history of MH. In addition to general questions about complications associated with previous surgeries and anesthesia, the patient should be asked if there has ever been an incident of unexplained high fever after anesthesia and if there are any muscular problems or diseases that run in the patient's family. Positive answers warrant in-depth investigation; previous medical records should be obtained, and the surgeon and anesthesia provider should be notified.

Medication history is especially important. Checklists for the patient to complete are helpful, as is the practice of having the patient bring all current medications if there is a preoperative visit. Over-the-counter medications are frequently not mentioned, but a recent U.S. epidemiologic study found that 87% of elderly individuals were taking at least one over-the-counter medication, and 6% of those questioned were taking five or more. With the increasing popularity of homeopathic and herbal medications, all adults should be specifically questioned about medications they purchase without a prescription, including aspirin and nonsteroidal anti-inflammatory drugs (NSAIDs) such as ibuprofen, which may cause clotting abnormalities. Additionally, the nurse should prompt the patient to try to remember all medication products they take such as patches, creams, eyedrops, inhalers, "shots," herbal or mineral supplements, and vitamins (Manno & Hayes, 2006).

Some vitamins and nutritional supplements, including vitamin E, fish oils and garlic, decrease platelet aggregation and increase bleeding times. Ideally, any supplement that may increase bleeding times should be discontinued a minimum of 1 week before surgery. The most dangerous herbal related perioperative events are bleeding, cardiovascular instability, or prolongation of anesthetic effect. The five most popular herbal supplements used in the United States are gingko biloba, St. John's wart, ginseng, garlic, and echinacea. All of these may produce adverse effects during surgery and anesthesia. The accepted guideline is to discontinue supplements with known adverse potential 2 to 3 weeks before surgery and selected diagnostic procedures, as well as not restarting them for at least 1 week after surgery (Ang-Lee, Yuan, & Moss, 2005). However, the hazards of abruptly discontinuing any supplement must be considered. Discontinuation could produce symptoms as when alcohol or narcotics are suddenly withdrawn. Currently, there is little definitive scientific information available, but, as an example, a possible dangerous situation could occur if St. John's Wort is suddenly discontinued. Because the herb is known to decrease the amount of other drugs and medications in the body, the concentrations of these substances could quickly rise to toxic levels.

Patients must be urged to be honest about substance abuse or recreational drug use. Explaining the dangerous consequences of not doing so may prove effective. For example, a patient who uses cocaine could suffer fatal dysrhythmias if the surgeon injects epinephrine, as in the use of a local anesthetic with epinephrine, during the procedure. Checklists or questionnaires tend to elicit more honest responses than direct questioning. Additionally, assuring patients that their answers are considered confidential and that questions are only asked to assure their personal safety may increase cooperation.

Medication reconciliation is a major focus in The Joint Commission's National Patient Safety Goals. Although there is continued controversy about the interpretation and implementation process for the medication standard, the intent is an important safety measure. On admission, during transfer to another caregiver and upon discharge, all the patient's medications should be reviewed in the context of other medications being administered or prescribed to avoid duplication or inadvertant adverse interactions.

Advocacy

The patient agreeing to ambulatory surgery assumes considerable responsibility for self-care. The patient and responsible adult who will attend him or her postoperatively must be capable of understanding and providing the level of care necessary. Discharging a patient into the care of a young adult the patient considers responsible, but who is not of legal age, may present a dilemma that should be resolved preoperatively. As the patient's advocate, the nurse should assist in arranging for preoperative assistance and postoperative care by community health care professionals if dependable friends or relatives are not available. Environmental factors should also be considered preoperatively. Distance from the facility to the home and available emergency treatment near the patient's home must be considered. Some ambulatory facilities arrange for an on-site interview in the patient's home allowing the nurse to evaluate and identify areas of postoperative concern. When this is not feasible, the nurse should try to identify potential postoperative living adjustments that may be necessary and stress to the patient and caregiver the need to make arrangements accordingly before the day of surgery.

As the patient's advocate, the nurse should discuss advance directives with the patient. This discussion is best done before the day of surgery to avoid upsetting the patient and to allow time for family discussion if appropriate. The nurse should be knowledgeable about the particular state's laws, be able to discuss various types of directives, and assist the patient in establishing a valid directive. If the patient has an advance directive, determine whether that directive speaks to the issue of resuscitation. Copies of the directive should be attached to the permanent medical record. Another responsibility of the nurse advocate is to note any signs of possible abuse and provide this information to the appropriate people or committee. The position statement of the American Society of PeriAnesthesia Nurses (ASPAN) (Table 2-2) provided the nurse with guidelines for addressing end-of-life issues with patients.

Informed Consent

Informed consent for surgery refers to voluntary consent given by a mentally competent prospective patient, or by a person legally responsible for the patient, for treatment after being informed of the purpose, methods, benefits, alternatives, and potential risks associated with the treatment. Awareness of risk is necessary for any person to make an informed choice.

The American College of Surgeons states in its Statements on Principles that "Patients should understand the indications for the operation, the risk involved, and the result that is hoped to attain." As part of their public information service, the college has suggested that every patient should ask his or her surgeon the following 10 questions before giving informed consent.

1. What are the indications that have led your doctor to the opinion that an operation is necessary?
2. What, if any, alternative treatments are available for your condition?
3. What will be the likely result if you don't have the operation?
4. What are the basic procedures involved in the operation?
5. What are the risks?
6. How is the operation expected to improve your health or quality of life?
7. Is hospitalization necessary and, if so, how long can you expect to be hospitalized?
8. What can you expect during your recovery period?
9. When can you expect to resume normal activities?
10. Are there likely to be residual effects from the operation?

(ACS, n.d.)

A major issue is the patient's capability of understanding the explanations; if the patient speaks a foreign language or is deaf, a qualified interpreter will be needed. Alternatives to the proposed treatment plan should also be presented. For a minor, consent is usually granted by the parent or legal guardian. Increasingly, older children are included in the decision-making process.

The ambulatory facility must have a legally approved consent form to document permission for staff members to provide patient care, which includes general treatment. General consent forms commonly include consent for anesthesia, but a separate process for and record of the patient's informed consent to anesthesia is recommended because a patient may allege that only the surgery, not the anesthesia, was discussed (Ireland, 1997).

After all details are explained to the patient by the surgeon and informed consent for the surgery is obtained, the perioperative nurse may obtain the patient's signature because there is a technical difference between consent and signing. Signing only

TABLE 2-2: A POSITION STATEMENT ON THE PERIANESTHESIA PATIENT WITH A DO-NOT-RESUSCITATE ADVANCE DIRECTIVE (1 OF 2)

Synopsis

Ethical care during the perianesthesia period requires that the nurse act in accordance with ethical principles and with a patient's predetermined end-of-life wishes. The perianesthesia nurse's ethical responsibilities encourage advocacy to assure a preanesthesia patient's consent is truly informed, autonomous and self-determined. The nurse also demonstrates respect by facilitating holistic concern for the perianesthesia patient's emotional, spiritual and educational well-being while providing physical safety.

A patient whose advance directive specifies no life sustaining measures may be unaware that cardiac or respiratory arrest are always potential yet usually reversible outcomes associated with anesthesia. When the patient's desires for the perianesthetic period are not specifically identified, anesthetic-related changes in physiologic function present the perianesthesia nurse with ethical conflict and confusion about appropriate interventions.

Background

1. An estimated 15% of surgical patients have an active do-not-resuscitate or do-not-intubate clause that reflects the elderly or chronically ill patient's considered preference for a "dignified death" without artificial life support.[1,2]
2. Palliative treatment, or comfort care or emergency events might require anesthesia and surgery. These interventions stress physiologic function, suppress consciousness, and precipitate transient, reversible decreases in cardiac and respiratory function, but are not associated with natural evolutions toward the patient's death.[2,3,4,5]
3. Applying endotracheal intubation and/or mechanical ventilation to support pulmonary function and medications or electric countershock to promote cardiac output are often specifically restricted in an advance directive document.[1,2,6,7] The patient and family may not be aware that these are usual interventions to support vital organ function during the perianesthesia period.
4. Ethically, ignoring the issue, assuming the patient's wishes or applying a facility policy or medical decision that automatically suspends any patient's Do-Not-Resuscitate (DNR)/Do-Not-Intubate (DNI) directive during the perioperative period denies the patient's right to self-determination and to autonomous, informed choices.[2,4,7,8]
5. The perianesthesia nurse is intimately involved in determining patient readiness for procedures, often is the "first-responder" who witnesses, then collaborates with physicians to intervene and evaluate the outcomes of respiratory and/or cardiac arrest.[3,4,6,11] Unclear communications and ambiguous or nonexistent facility policies about a patient's DNR/DNI status during the perianesthesia period do not direct and support a nurse's decisions and actions. Ethically, this nurse must choose between not responding, thereby doing harm (maleficence), and a professional and legal obligation to preserve life without harm (beneficence). These choices may conflict with the patient's stated end-of-life choices.[9,10,12]

Position

The American Society of PeriAnesthesia Nurses (ASPAN) recommends that at the time of surgery and prior to receiving any anesthetic medication, a patient with an active do-not-resuscitate advance directive must reconsider this designation and reclarify wishes about resuscitation during the perianesthetic period.

- To limit potential for ethical dilemmas, the patient's informed consent will include discussion of the advance directive, living will or physician order that specifies DNR or DNI during a candid and well-documented conversation with physicians and appropriate significant other(s).
- Each facility establishes and communicates a policy that identifies resources and procedures that detail the management of a patient's DNR/DNI status during the perianesthesia period.

Approval of Statement

This statement was approved by a vote of the ASPAN Board of Directors on April 20, 1996 in Phoenix, Arizona.

ASPAN joins other professional colleagues, specifically the American Nurses Association (ANA), the Association of Operating Room Nurses (AORN) and the American Society of Anesthesiologists (ASA), in considering the ethical implications of the advance directive.

A Glossary of Commonly used Ethics Terminology

Principles: Guidelines for Decisions:

I. **Autonomy:** A patient's right to self-determination. Respect for autonomy is considered the primary, fundamental guide to ethical decision-making and supersedes other values.

TABLE 2-2: A POSITION STATEMENT ON THE PERIANESTHESIA PATIENT WITH A DO-NOT-RESUSCITATE ADVANCE DIRECTIVE (2 OF 2)

i. Includes truth-telling (veracity), freedom and right to information.

ii. Inhibited by paternalism or "deciding for" another; imposing the beliefs of another (nurse, physician, family member) onto the patient, eliminating the right to choose.

II. **Nonmaleficence:** the expectation that interventions will "do no harm." Balances risk in relation to benefit.

III. **Beneficence:** the intention to "do good." Includes compassion and respect for persons and actions in the patient's best interests.

IV. **Fidelity:** faithfulness in relationship to others. Includes upholding professional obligations.

V. **Justice:** fair resource allocation, including benefits and burdens of equitable access to care.

Values: Basis for Nursing Actions:

I. **Advocacy:** maintain awareness of issues, policies and channels to help secure the interests of a patient.

II. **Competence:** maintain current nursing knowledge related to the field of practice.

III. **Caring:** intentional empathy and acting from an internal source of compassion to benefit another. Includes respect for persons, honesty, privacy and confidentiality.

Definitions:

I. **Do-Not-Resuscitate order:** specific physician order on a medical record that specifies no cardiopulmonary resuscitation. Includes intubation and cardiac support.

I. **Advance directive:** a written legal document initiated by a competent individual that specifies this person's wishes for health care interventions. Enacted at some future time when the individual becomes unable to decide or express wishes. Includes a living will and/or a durable power of attorney for health care.

References with Annotations

1. Clemency, MV, Thompson, NJ. "Do not resuscitate" (DNR) orders and the anesthesiologist: A survey... Anesth Analg. 1993, 76:394-401. After surveying anesthesiologists Anesth Analg to determine opinions and experience with DNR orders during the perianesthetic period, authors recommend discussion to define issues, clear confusion and, with patients, mutually determine actions. In this survey, over 60% assumed a DNR order should be suspended and most do not discuss plans to intubate or resuscitate.

2. Marigolis, JO, McGrath, MJ, Kussin, PS, et al. Do not resuscitate (DNR) orders during surgery: ethical foundations for institutional policies in the United States. Anesth Analg. 1995, 80:806-809. Authors present dimensions of ethical decision-making, suggest four approaches to manage DNR orders for the perianesthetic period, then recommend that each facility develop a policy addressing the issue and presenting options to patients.

3. Curtin, LL. DNR in the OR: Ethical considerations and hospital policies. Nurs Manag. 1994, 25(2):29-31. Editorial that identifies ethical and legal aspects of perioperative DNR is a dimension of informed consent and perhaps as responsible, informative (and easy) as providing postoperative instructions. Reminds readers that nurses need only to respond to the questions and issues, not provide answers.

4. Jacobsen, DS. Ethical dilemmas of do-not-resuscitate orders in surgery. AORN Jour. 1994, 60(3):449-452 Promotes frank discussion with patients, then individualizing decisions about DNR orders during the perioperative period. Identifies ethical dilemmas, principles and values related to these discussions.

5. Association of Operating Room Nurses. Position statement on perioperative care of patients with do-not-resuscitate (DNR) orders. AORN Jour. 1995, 61(1):60. Presents the proposal of AORN's position and rationale for considering this topic.

Igoe, S, Cascella, S, Stockdale, K. Ethics in the OR: DNR and Patient Autonomy. Nurs Manag. 1993, 24(9):112A,112S,112H. Discusses the role of the facility ethics committee to address ethical and procedural concerns related to a patient's DNR status during the perioperative period. Advocating for patient autonomy respects informed consent and self-determination.

6. Cohen, CB, Cohen, PJ. Required reconsideration of "do-not-resuscitate" orders in the operating room and certain other treatment settings. Law, Med & Hlth Care. 1992, 20:354-363. Promotes abandoning facility-wide DNR policies in favor of policy that requires that a patient's DNR directive be reconsidered for the perioperative period.

7. Truog, RD. "Do-not-resuscitate" orders during anesthesia and surgery. Anesthesiology. 1991, 74:606-608. Recommends abandoning rigid policies that require perioperative suspension of DNR orders. Consider guidelines and a practice of responding "individually and compassionately" to resolve ethical conflicts.

8. American Nurses Association. Code for nurses. Washington, DC: ANA; 1995 Fundamental document that underlies nursing's professional responsibilities to patients, including respect for dignity, right to privacy, accountability for actions competence, integrity and responsibility for standards of practice.

9. American Nurses Association. Compendium of position statements on the nurse's role in end-of-life decisions. Washington, DC: ANA; 1992. A collection of ANA's established positions on a variety of topics related to end-of-life decisions. Includes assisted suicide and do-not-resuscitate decisions.

10. Keffer, MJ, Keffer, HL. The do-not-resuscitate order: moral responsibilities of the perioperative nurse. AORN Jour. 1994, 59(3):641-650. Recommends nursing familiarity with perioperative patient care policies and willingness to advocate for the patient amid conflicts related to DNR decisions. Article identifies ethical concerns and nursing responsibilities.

11. Rothenberg, DM. Ethical considerations for cardiopulmonary resuscitation. Anesth Clinics of North Amer. 1995, 13(4):999-1016. Discusses CPR research and ethical considerations related to decisions about resuscitation to prevent futile efforts to resuscitate organs that are "too weak to live."

documents that earlier consent was given (Ireland, 1997). However, if the patient is unwilling or seems uninformed about the proposed procedure, the nurse should not have the consent signed and should notify the surgeon. Ambulatory surgery facilities may be responsible for validating that the consent process has been conducted to the patient's satisfaction (Darwin Professional Underwriters Inc., 2006). In addition, the signature must be obtained before any medication is administered.

Similarly, for patients who refuse the use of blood transfusion or the use of blood products, such as Jehovah's Witnesses, or those who designate and limit donors to family members, a signed and witnessed blood refusal form or document stating the patient's wishes should be obtained and made a permanent part of the chart, even for minor outpatient procedures (Darwin Professional Underwriters Inc., 2006). Additional special situations that require informed consent include students performing or participating in any procedure; the presence of equipment manufacturing representatives or other nonemployees; taking photographs, videotaping, or producing slides of a procedure; procedures for the disposal of tissue or its use in grafts; or any procedure that is experimental, including clinical trials or institutional review board consents (Darwin Professional Underwriters Inc., 2006).

Patient Rights

In December 1991, the Patient Self-Determination Act (PSDA) became effective, stipulating that individuals receiving medical care be given written information about their rights, according to the laws of their state of residence, in order to make informed decisions about that care. This information includes the right to accept or refuse medical or surgical care. The act also specifies the right to initiate advance directives, such as living wills and durable power of attorney (Berrio & Levesque, 1996). Thereafter, many states enacted consumer protection laws relative to managed care. Recognizing the importance of protecting the privacy of health information because of the rapid evolution of health information systems, congress passed the Health Insurance Portability and Accountability Act (HIPAA), which became law in August, 1996.

The following year, President Clinton created the Advisory Commission on Consumer Protection and Quality in the Health Care Industry that developed a Patient's Bill of Rights, the principles of which have been adopted by many health plans. Additionally, the Office for Civil Rights enforces the federal law that protects the privacy of health information along with civil rights in health care and social services. Congress passed a Patient's Bill of Rights in 2001, but it was vetoed by President George W. Bush.

The American Hospital Association (AHA) published a Patient's Bill of Rights based on a foundation of respect for human beings as individuals and emphasizing active patient participation in decisions about the care they will receive (Messner & Lewis, 1996). Twelve rights are discussed in detail, yet the first states simply that "The patient has a right to considerate and respectful care."

The Joint Commission also affirms that patients' rights and personal dignity should be respected and care should be based on individual needs. It also addresses the right of the patient to make decisions affecting care.

Although variables affecting patient satisfaction may differ among age and cultural groups (Yellen, 2003) individuals' satisfaction is directly related to considerate and respectful care. A survey of nearly 140,000 patients identified 15 major indicators of patient satisfaction, most of which involved basic rights and quality communication. The number one indicator involved staff concern for the patient's privacy (Messner & Lewis, 1996).

However, patients also have responsibilities, including the responsibility to provide information

Porphyria - a group of rare disorders, passed down thru families, in which important part of Hgb, called heme is not made properly. Heme is also found in myoglobin a protein found in certain muscles.

about previous medical and surgical care, to follow the instructions given by the physician and of other patients, and to provide information to the health care facility about the ability to pay for services. Facilities commonly develop printed information about rights and responsibilities for distribution to their specific patient populations.

Anesthetic Assessment

The preoperative assessment by the anesthesia provider is meant to build on, not duplicate, the nursing assessment for the procedure. A skilled perioperative nurse may identify areas of concern and provide valuable information to facilitate safe anesthetic management; especially if the patient is not seen by the anesthesia provider prior to the day of surgery. When there is a positive or suggested history of previous anesthetic complications or allergic reactions, a review of previous records is warranted if they can be obtained. It is also important that the anesthetic history of blood relatives be evaluated because genetic predisposition is associated with potential anesthetic complications, such as MH, porphyria, and low plasma cholinesterase (pseudocholinesterase) levels that prolong response to succinylcholine.

Medications and substances of all types that the patient may be taking are often unreported but are very important to anesthetic management. Researchers at the Tulane University School of Medicine conducted a survey asking surgical patients, after their preoperative examination, to circle all listed medications they were taking. The list included antidepressants, antipsychotics, benzodiazepines, lithium, and over-the-counter drugs known to affect mood, such as insomnia remedies containing melatonin. Forty-three percent of the patients scheduled for elective surgery were taking one or more of these medications (Scher, 1998). Patients may become annoyed when asked the same questions by different people, so it is important to inform the patient at the beginning of care that many people will likley be asking the same question and that it is not because the staff does not document or share the proper information. Rather it is because they are continually checking to be sure they provide safe care. The medical record should be carefully reviewed for the patient's medical history, physical examination findings, results of diagnostic procedures and tests, and pertinent personal information. All information should be evaluated relative to how it may impact the patient's response to and need for anesthesia. The patient is then interviewed and examined, addressing specific areas of concern and importance.

A major area of concern is airway maintenance during the procedure or in the event of an emergency situation. Previous head or neck surgery, radiation therapy, chronic neck pain, hoarseness, or sleep apnea are important considerations. The general state of dentition should be examined and documented, including loose teeth, missing teeth, protruding incisors, chipped or cracked teeth, partial and full dentures, crowns, and other cosmetic dental prostheses. Mobility of the jaw and neck, including extension capability of the neck, also should be examined. Joint mobility may also be evaluated, and complaints of pain or limitation of motion should be noted on the medical record to establish a reference for comparison if postoperative complaints develop. This information is also helpful for protective intra-operative positioning. If regional anesthesia is anticipated, the site of injection should be examined for anomalies or skin infection. Potential venous access difficulties also should be noted. The choice of anesthetic agents and technique is influenced by the type of surgery, the patient's physical status, the patient's preference, and the surgeon's preference. As with the surgical procedure, the options, techniques, benefits, and risks should be discussed with the patient or legal guardian, and a plan should be developed for anesthetic management. When all questions have been clearly answered and the patient agrees to the plan, legal consent is obtained.

Preanesthesia Clinics

The need for proper preanesthesia workup before ambulatory surgery has prompted establishment of preanesthesia clinics. Here patients have their history and physical done, have necessary diagnostic tests performed, and receive perioperative education and consultation. In the preanesthesia clinic the patient is seen by the anesthesia provider, who has the opportunity to identify patients at risk, plan appropriate anesthetic and postanesthetic care, provide patient education, and develop a rapport with the patient. Registration and paperwork necessary for admission to the ambulatory facility is also completed. Although there are costs involved for a preanesthesia clinic, they are offset because of the significant reductions in preoperative laboratory tests, consultations, and operating room turnover time, and canceled operations (Pandit, 1999).

Some ASCs, particularly those affiliated with hospitals, are utilizing nurse practitioners (NPs) to conduct patient preoperative assessments. These primary care NPs practice in an outpatient setting in a hospital environment in accordance with the particular mandates of the individual state (Guida, 2004).

Major NP goals in this setting are to evaulate patients without a primary care physician or who are unable to be seen by their physicians appropriately and chart readiness prior to surgery, thus preventing delays or cancellations. Should previously unrecognized health concerns, such as hypertension, be found, the surgeon may be notified for appropriate preoperative treatment. For all patients seen, the NP conducts a detailed assessment, incorporating the topics discussed in this chapter. Patient education and psychological support are important roles of the NP affiliated with an ASC (Guida, 2004).

Depending on the particular state's Advanced Practice Nursing Board, the NP serving an ASC may work under a collaborative practice with an appropriate physician. Usually, the NP and ASC staff interaction is limited to preadmission staff and the nurse manager. Although not normally involved with the perianesthesia staff, ASPAN recommends that the NP be certified as a postanesthesia nurse or an ambulatory perianesthesia nurse (ASPAN, 1996).

PATIENT EDUCATION

Every interaction between the perioperative nurse and the patient and his or her family, or caregiver, is a teaching opportunity. Patient teaching is especially important in ambulatory surgery because of the self-care responsibilities assumed when the patient agrees to have a procedure done on an outpatient basis. Family members and caregivers must be included in the educational process to prepare them to assume responsibility for care normally provided by health care professionals in hospital settings. In addition to reducing anxiety, effective patient education is known to increase self-esteem by increasing self-efficacy, decrease perceived pain postoperatively, and speed recovery (Fox, 1998). Preparing patients and their families for the procedure and management of their postoperative recovery and convalescence is important to improving satisfaction and outcomes (Zanchetta & Bernstein, 2004).

For learning to occur, the timing and setting must be conducive to learning, and the learner (patient) must be receptive. A patient overwhelmed with anxiety, worries, or pain is not receptive to learning. When these concerns have been addressed, learning and retention are more likely to take place.

Face-to-face interviews before the day of surgery, when the patient is less anxious, are most effective for eliciting information and teaching (Dunn, 1998), but when this interaction is not possible a well-conducted telephone interview and conversation at least 1 to 2 days before admission is essential for preoperative instruction. However, beyond what to expect intraoperatively and postoperatively, studies polling patient opinions have shown that patients feel that learning new skills for postoperative care is best provided after admission to the ambulatory surgery facility (Fox, 1998). (See Chapter 5.)

Studies have shown that patients who ask questions and want to be well informed have lower levels of preoperative stress and more effective problem-focused coping strategies. Preference for information usually is significantly and negatively correlated with level of education.

The material must be presented at the learner's level of understanding. Knowing the patient's prior medical history and type of employment, along with assessing the educational level, may provide insights to the patient's ability to understand abstract or complex concepts. Evaluation of the patient's comprehension may be possible by posing questions to the patient and requesting return demonstration. However, if the patient is unable to fully understand the information due to language or culture his or her well-being may be jeopardized rather than benefited. Language and cultural assistance result in a patient more likely to participate in his or her recovery and have a better surgical experience. Communication with the patient should include provision of education and training appropriate to the individual's needs, abilities, learning preferences, and readiness to learn.

Methods of teaching common to ambulatory settings include one-on-one conversation; demonstration, practice, and return demonstration; visual aids such as videotapes that can be viewed in the facility or taken home; and written material for the patient's review and reference.

Common preoperative learning needs for the ambulatory patient include

- what will be done in preparation for the procedure;
- what they must do the evening before and the day of the procedure;
- what type of postoperative support must be available in the home;
- what they may experience at the facility, including sights, sounds, and sensations.

Typically, the perioperative nurse provides most patient and caregiver teaching and support, but providing in-depth information on the surgical procedure or speculation on the results or complications is not the role of the nurse. The physician should explain why the surgery is necessary, how it will be performed, the potential benefits and risks, and any diagnostic pre-procedure testing required.

The day before surgery, the patient should be contacted to review the preoperative instructions. Having the patient or caregiver verbally repeat, describe, or demonstrate the written instructions provides the opportunity to assess the understanding. Patients with language difficulties or those unable to read may try to avoid this step, which should alert the caller that compliance may be questionable. The nurse should repeat the instructions slowly and simply and have the patient repeat them.

Patients need preoperative instructions regarding medications they take for existing medical conditions. Unless ordered otherwise, most cardiovascular, asthma, antihypertensive, and anticonvulsant therapy is generally continued until the time of surgery. Medication for Parkinson's disease is also usually continued until surgery and resumed as soon as the patient is able to tolerate oral ingestion postoperatively. All medication instructions should be on the orders of the physician.

The type of anesthesia the patient will receive may be an important factor in whether or not hypertensive medication is discontinued before surgery. Angiotensin-converting enzyme inhibitors such as captopril (Capoten) and enalapril (Vasotec) may be withheld to avoid adverse reaction during general anesthesia induction and tracheal intubation. Conversely, betablockers and clonidine (Catapres) should be taken with a small amount of water the day of surgery to avoid rebound hypertension, myocardial ischemia, or severe dysrhythmias (Smith, Muir, & Hall, 1996). Asthmatic patients should be told to bring their bronchodilator inhaler with them the day of surgery because the medication may be necessary to treat breathing difficulty related to anxiety or to lessen the possibility of coughing or bronchospasm during induction of general anesthesia.

Anticoagulants are usually stopped several days before surgery to allow the prothrombin time to return to normal. If a patient receiving MAO inhibitor therapy is deemed suitable for ambulatory surgery, it is no longer recommended that the therapy be discontinued before anesthesia. However, meperidine (Demerol) and ephedrine should be avoided in patients receiving MAO inhibitor therapy (Long, 1997). Newer antidepressants, such as selective serotonin reuptake inhibitors (SSRIs), should also be continued perioperatively because abrupt withdrawal may result in untoward symptoms. Meperidine, pentazocine, and tramadol should not be used with SSRIs (Golembiewski, 2006). Patients with insulin-controlled diabetes will need an individualized preoperative and postoperative regimen. Patients should also be advised that any oral medication required the morning of surgery should be taken with one sip of water. Explaining why something must be done or will be done is usually better than presenting lists of do's and don'ts. For example, explaining that the concept of nothing-by-mouth (NPO) is a safety feature to prevent serious complications may enhance compliance. Explaining that, in addition to no food or liquid intake, NPO includes not chewing gum or sucking on lozenges because either may stimulate the production of gastric acid.

Patient understanding facilitates patient compliance. The nurse should make sure the patient clearly understands:

- when to begin the NPO countdown – specifically by hour, rather than "6 hours before."
- when to arrive at the ambulatory surgical center – again, the specific hour.
- what to leave at home – jewelry, valuables and cosmetic prostheses if appropriate. (To promote safety and reduce stress, glasses and hearing aids may be worn and removed before receiving medication or undergoing surgery. This action should be documented, and the items should be placed in safekeeping. Contact lenses must be removed.)
- what to wear – loose-fitting clothes, low-heeled shoes.
- what to bring – insurance card and any necessary co-pay.
- required durable medical equipment such as crutches or walker.

When communicating with the patient, the nurse should always explain and never assume.

Discharge planning and postoperative teaching also begin preoperatively (Dunn, 1998; Watkins & White, 2001; Kamming et al., 2004; Pasero & Belden, 2006). Patients' self-care for postdischarge symptoms depends on information provided by the nurse during the preoperative interview, then again before discharge (Fetzer, Hand, Bouchard, Smith, & Jenkins, 2005). The nurse doing the preoperative assessment should discuss postoperative restrictions so the patient can plan ahead for work and home responsibilities. It should be made clear that, depending on the nature of the surgery, there may be an extended recovery period. The amount, quality, and probable duration of postoperative discomfort to be reasonably expected must be presented carefully and diplomatically to inform not alarm. Pain is less likely to be distressing when it is expected (Doyle, 1999). Preconceived expectations based on hearsay need to be dispelled or clarified.

Studies have shown that providing patients with valid information about what they are likely to experience, including the expected level of discomfort, decreases pain experienced and analgesic use.

Similarly, information related to physiologic coping, such as coughing, deep breathing, turning, and ambulation also reduces the need for pain medication.

Just as obtaining an oxygen saturation level preoperatively aids in evaluating the patient during the postsurgery recovery phase, obtaining a preoperative pain profile aids in postoperative evaluation and treatment of pain. Information elicited from the patient or caregiver should include:

- significant previous or ongoing instances of pain and its effect on the patient
- previously used methods for pain control that the patient has found either helpful or not helpful
- the patient's attitude toward the use of opioid, sedative, or other medications, including any history of substance abuse
- the patient's typical coping response for stress or pain, including the possible presence of disorders such as depression, anxiety, or psychosis
- family expectations and beliefs regarding pain, stress, and postoperative course
- ways the patient describes and shows pain
- patient knowledge of, and preferences for, pain management methods and instruction.

During the preoperative assessment, the patient should be given practical advice about pain management at home. Just before discharge on the day of surgery this information should be reinforced verbally and in writing for the patient and caregiver (Doyle, 1999). It is important for the patient and caregiver to understand that it is more effective to prevent pain than to treat it once it has been established.

SUMMARY

Preoperative assessment is a time for learning and instructing. The nurse should learn as much about the patient's history and current condition as possible, and instruct the patient on how best to prepare for surgery, experience the ambulatory procedure, and cope postoperatively. To successfully accomplish these objectives, the nurse should not overlook the need to support the patient psychologically.

Again, ambulatory surgery patients should be assessed as thoroughly as a hospitalized patient would be, relative to the surgical procedure and patient's physical and mental condition. The family should be included whenever appropriate.

EXAM QUESTIONS

CHAPTER 2

Questions 10-17

Note: Choose the option that BEST answers each question.

10. A surgical procedure may be considered unsuitable for an outpatient if it
    a. requires postoperative analgesia.
    b. requires a pneumatic tourniquet.
    c. involves major blood loss.
    d. involves a lower extremity.

11. Optimal perioperative management and favorable outcomes are most dependent upon
    a. patient compliance.
    b. thorough preoperative assessment.
    c. interdepartmental communication.
    d. resources of the facility.

12. By arranging for preoperative or postdischarge assistance needed by the patient, the nurse is acting as the
    a. team manager.
    b. organizational developer.
    c. quality assurer.
    d. patient's advocate.

13. A statement indicating the patient understands the nature of the surgery, as well as the risks and benefits, is considered
    a. due process.
    b. informed consent.
    c. Medicare compatible.
    d. facility specific.

14. A separate signed consent is recommended for
    a. IV medications.
    b. laparoscopic procedures.
    c. early discharge.
    d. anesthesia.

15. If the patient has major questions or misunderstandings about the scheduled procedure, the perioperative nurse should
    a. explain risks as clearly as possible.
    b. explain the procedure as clearly as possible.
    c. withhold medications and notify the surgeon.
    d. administer medications but notify the surgeon.

16. Consent for treatment must be signed by the patient
    a. when the operating physician is present.
    b. before any medication is administered.
    c. in the presence of two witnesses.
    d. in duplicate.

17. Self-care responsibilities being assumed by the ambulatory surgical patient and caregivers increases the need for
    a. home-health care personnel.
    b. delayed discharge.
    c. information and instruction.
    d. access to a cellular phone.

CHAPTER 3

ANESTHETIC MANAGEMENT

CHAPTER OBJECTIVE

Upon completion of this chapter, the reader will be able to recognize anesthetic agents and techniques and the applicability and appropriateness of each for ambulatory surgical procedures.

LEARNING OBJECTIVES

Upon completion of this chapter, the reader will be able to

1. discriminate between general, regional, and local anesthesia.
2. recognize the anesthetic agents used to produce each type of anesthesia.
3. identify the techniques used to produce each type of anesthesia.
4. describe nursing care considerations for each type of anesthesia.

INTRODUCTION

Because patients about to undergo ambulatory surgery tend to be concerned about pain and awareness during surgery, yet are equally apprehensive about being given anesthesia, it is important that the perioperative nurse be knowledgeable about the anesthetic process. An understanding of that process will enhance patient care preoperatively, intraoperatively, and postoperatively. The intent of this chapter is to provide a concise but comprehensive basic understanding of anesthetic management for ambulatory surgery.

PREMEDICATION

The emphasis for anesthesia given for ambulatory surgery is on achieving "home readiness" as safely and quickly as possible. Controversy exists over the use of sedative and analgesic premedication in an outpatient setting, owing to their possible prolongation of recovery time.

Primary objectives of premedication are relief of anxiety and some degree of sedation. Ideally, any medication prescribed for outpatients should have rapid onset of action and should not prolong recovery nor unduly impair psychomotor skills. Unfortunately, most sedatives, hypnotics, and analgesics currently available impair psychomotor performance. Coordination and fine motor skills may be impaired for up to 12 hours. However, preoperative anxiety, stress, and postoperative pain also interfere with postoperative psychomotor function. Table 3-1 summarizes the different classifications of preoperative medications.

Benzodiazepines

Oral benzodiazepines are popular choices as premedications. Midazolam (Versed) is a potent amnesic and anxiolytic rapidly absorbed from the gastrointestinal tract, with peak plasma concentra-

TABLE 3-1: PREOPERATIVE MEDICATIONS

CLASSIFICATION	USE	EXAMPLES
Tranquilizers	Antianxiety, sedation	**Benzodiazepines:** midazolam (Versed), diazepam (Valium), lorazepam (Ativan)
	Antiemetic	**Phenothiazines:** hydroxyzine (Vistaril), promethazine (Phenergan) **Butyrophenones:** droperidol (Inapsine)
Opioids	Analgesia, sedation	Morphine, meperidine (Demerol), fentanyl (Sublimaze)
Opioids agonist-antagonist	Analgesia, sedation	Nalbuphine (Nubain), butorphanol (Stadol)
Barbiturates	Sedation	Pentobarbital (Nembutal), secobarbital (Seconal)
Anticholinergics	Reduction of tracheobronchial and oral secretions, bradycardia	**Belladonna compounds:** atropine, scopolamine (transdermal scopolamine may also produce antiemetic effect)
	Reduction of vagal reflexes	**Synthetic:** glycopyrrolate (Robinul)
Gastrokinetic dopamine antagonist	Aspiration prophylaxis Acceleration of gastric emptying Antiemetic	Metoclopramide (Reglan)
5-HT_3 receptor blocking agents	Antiemetic	Ondansetron (Zofran) Dolasetron (Anzemet)
Histamine-2 receptor antagonists	Aspiration prophylaxis Suppression of gastric acid secretion	Cimetidine (Tagamet), ranitidine (Zantac), famotidine (Pepcid)
Antacids Clear, nonparticulate	Aspiration prophylaxis Buffer gastric acid	Sodium citrate (Bicitra), sodium citrate with potassium citrate (Polycitra)

tion and corresponding clinical effects generally occurring within 1 hour. Because of extensive first-pass hepatic extraction, only 40% to 50% of orally administered midazolam reaches the systemic circulation. Consequently, an oral dose of midazolam must be approximately twice that of an intravenous (IV) dose to achieve comparable effects.

Midazolam exhibits a short half-life, but its rapid disappearance from the bloodstream does not guarantee fast recovery. Instead, recovery may be similar to diazepam (Valium), which has been shown to affect coordination and reaction skills for up to 5 hours. This lack of correlation between half-life and clinical recovery has also been found when IV midazolam and diazepam are compared in sedative techniques.

However, when used as premedications, moderate oral doses of midazolam do not adversely affect the quality and duration of recovery after brief general anesthetic exposures, whereas small doses may fail to produce sufficient relief from anxiety. Small and moderate doses of oral midazolam may result in significantly impaired performance for at least 2 hours after surgery. Dizziness is also a potential side effect of benzodiazepines, regardless of the dosage.

Benzodiazepines are available in liquid form for children, but midazolam has an unpleasant taste so it is best given with a small amount of a sweet liquid other than fruit juice, which may affect the medication's metabolism.

Opioid Analgesics

The use of opioid analgesics as premedications in an ambulatory surgery setting is controversial. Although it seems advisable to avoid the use of long-acting narcotics, the use of fentanyl (Sublimaze) or sufentanil (Sufenta) may decrease the sedative-hypnotic medication requirements intraoperatively. Postoperative nausea and vomiting frequently associated with opioids may prolong recovery.

Patients who receive short-acting narcotics and do not experience undesirable side effects may have a more rapid recovery than do patients who receive benzodiazepines because of the lower doses of anesthetic required intraoperatively. Outpatients undergoing procedures associated with significant postoperative pain may benefit from the use of longer acting narcotics, which may provide effective analgesia after discharge.

For particularly anxious patients who might benefit from preoperative pharmacologic support, the sparing and judicious use of benzodiazepines or short-acting opioid analgesics may be advisable. This approach may be especially applicable for patients undergoing regional anesthesia (i.e., regional block) when, despite skin infiltration of the injection site with a local anesthetic, there may be discomfort during the placement of the block.

Innovative methods of administration are available for patients unable or unwilling to take oral premedication but requiring medication before an IV is started. Fentanyl has been shown to be effectively absorbed transmucosally in lollipop form (oral transmucosal fentanyl citrate) and provides a pleasant, nonthreatening method of delivering preanesthetic medication, especially to children. Onset of action occurs within 5 to 15 minutes, with maximum reduction in apprehension and peak analgesic effect seen 20 to 30 minutes after the start of administration. Because only approximately 25% to 33% of the total dose is absorbed by the oral mucosa, while the remainder is swallowed and is slowly absorbed from the gastrointestinal tract, the actual bioavailability of the total dosage of transmucosal fentanyl is approximately 50% (Brislin & Rose, 2005).

Antiemetics and Aspiration Prophylaxis

Certain physiologic conditions predispose the patient to regurgitation of gastric contents, possibly resulting in pulmonary aspiration. Examples of such conditions include morbid obesity, hiatal hernia with reflux, pregnancy, and diabetes. Extreme anxiety, fear, and use of opioids are additional risk factors. These patients may benefit from the preoperative administration of antiemetics. Combining agents with different modes of action may increase efficacy.

Metoclopramide (Reglan) is a gastrokinetic medication with central and peripheral actions. It increases motility of the upper gastrointestinal tract and accelerates gastric emptying. Metoclopramide may be administered orally, IV, or intramuscularly (IM), either prophylactically as a preoperative medication or as a postoperative treatment for nausea. It has no sedative effect, but dystonia or other extrapyramidal effects are possible, especially with the concurrent use of phenothiazines or butyrophenones (e.g., droperidol) that also have antinausea effects.

Anticholinergic medications such as atropine sulfate and glycopyrrolate (Robinul) block the gastrointestinal effects of metoclopramide. Metoclopramide decreases the absorption of orally administered cimetidine and decreases dosage requirements of the ultra short-acting barbiturate induction agent thiopental (Pentothal) (Morgan, Mikhail, & Murray, 2006).

Ondansetron (Zofran) is a selective serotonin 5-HT_3 receptor antagonist that acts centrally in the brain and peripherally at vagal nerve endings. Unlike metoclopramide, it does not affect gastrointestinal motility but appears to play an important role in initiation of the vomiting reflex (Morgan,

Mikhail, & Murray, 2006). Ondansetron has no sedative effect and may be given either orally or by IV; pain may be experienced with IV injection.

A study of optimal timing for the administration of ondansetron as a prophylactic antiemetic in ambulatory settings found that administering ondansetron by IV immediately before the end of surgery was the most efficacious method of preventing postoperative nausea and vomiting, facilitating early recovery and improving patient satisfaction (Tang et al., 1998).

Dolasetron (Anzemet), a 5-HT_3 receptor blocking antiemetic agent, may cause prolongation of cardiac conduction intervals. It should be used cautiously or avoided in patients on anti-arrhythmic medications, high dose anthracycline therapy, or diuretics that may cause electrolyte imbalance such as hypokalemia.

Histamine-2 (H_2)-receptor antagonists cimetidine (Tagamet), ranitidine (Zantac), and famotidine (Pepcid) inhibit gastric acid secretion. They may be given orally or by IV, preferably at bedtime the evening before surgery and repeated at least 2 hours before surgery. H_2-receptor antagonists only affect the pH of gastric acids secreted after their administration.

Bicitra or *Polycitra,* nonparticulate antacids, are given by mouth just before surgery but are thought to lose their effectiveness 30 to 60 minutes after ingestion. Nonparticulate antacids are less damaging to the alveoli of the lung if aspirated than are particulate antacids such as aluminum or magnesium hydroxide (Morgan, Mikhail, & Murray, 2006). However, they do increase gastric volume.

Application of a transdermal scopolamine patch 2 hours before surgery may be effective for nausea, but the anticholinergic side effects associated with scopolamine, such as dry mouth, blurred vision, disorientation, and urinary retention, may be a contraindication.

GENERAL ANESTHESIA

Anesthesia means loss of sensation. It may be produced in a small, localized area of the body (local anesthesia), in a particular region of the body (regional anesthesia) or, with sufficient pharmacologically induced depression of the cerebral cortex, a state of controlled unconsciousness with loss of sensation (general anesthesia) may be achieved. Under adequate general anesthesia, the patient is unable to maintain control of the airway or respond purposefully to external stimulation.

The ambulatory surgery setting presents the anesthesia care provider with challenges and concerns beyond those for inpatient surgery. In addition to being awake, breathing spontaneously, being stable physiologically, and being able to respond to instruction, the ambulatory patient recovering from surgery must, in a short period of time, be able to walk safely, take fluids without vomiting, void, understand and remember instructions, and be able to take oral pain medication. To achieve these goals, the anesthetic plan typically involves the use of a combination of fast-acting IV and inhalation agents.

Factors Influencing the Use of General Anesthesia

Circumstances that may contribute to the choice of a general anesthetic technique include:

- *Patient age and mental status* – extremes of age or the inability to cooperate may complicate the procedure.
- *Requirements of the surgery*

  Duration – may exceed the duration of regional block or local infiltration that can be achieved using therapeutic doses of appropriate anesthetics.

  Position – may be too restrictive and uncomfortable for patient to tolerate.

  Muscular relaxation – may require the use of neuromuscular blocking agents (NMBAs) that will affect the patient's ability to breathe spontaneously.

- *Patient preference* – patients sometimes refuse to undergo a surgical procedure if they are not completely unconscious. This response is usually due to fear, including fear of paralysis from a regional block or a previous unsatisfactory anesthetic experience.

The anesthesia provider also makes the decision about the appropriateness of general anesthesia by evaluating potential contraindications, either absolute or relative. The patient's physical and diagnostic assessment may uncover unstable metabolic, cardiac or respiratory diseases that need to be considered. Contraindications to general anesthesia include:

- *Full stomach* – implies the danger of regurgitation of gastric contents into the hypopharynx with subsequent aspiration into the lungs. Regurgitation may be passive by reflux or active due to vomiting. In an outpatient setting, a full stomach is usually due to the patient's failure to follow preoperative fasting instructions (NPO status).
- *Physical status* – reimbursement issues are mandating that more procedures be performed on an outpatient basis, which can increase the likelihood of patients with poorly controlled systemic disease (class P3 and P4 risks) presenting for ambulatory surgery.
- *Abnormal preoperative test results that may affect the anesthesia provider's decision*:
  - low hematocrit or hemoglobin, which will affect the oxygen carrying power of the red blood cells
  - unstable heart rate indicated by electrocardiogram (ECG)
  - chest pathology
  - compromised hepatic or urinary status.
- *Upper respiratory infection* (URI) – increased secretions may cause coughing and laryngospasm, compromised ventilation, and spreading of infection.

Progression of Anesthesia

Traditionally, the progression of anesthesia is defined by four stages: I – analgesia, II – delirium, III – surgical anesthesia, IV – medullary depression. Stage III is further divided into four planes. All of these stages and planes may be achieved and observed if the sole anesthetic administered is an inhalation agent, as used for young children. However, with the use of ultra short-acting IV barbiturates and sedative-hypnotics, stages I and II pass so quickly that they are not readily observable. For this reason, general anesthesia is more practically divided into induction, maintenance, and recovery.

General anesthesia may be induced with the use of an ultra short-acting IV agent, an inhalation anesthetic, or a combination of these, until the level of surgical anesthesia is achieved. During the maintenance phase, the depth of anesthesia is adjusted as necessary based on surgical progress and patient response.

Although unconscious, a patient at a light level of anesthesia may respond adversely to surgical stimulation (or other external stimulation). This response may manifest as an increase in blood pressure, an increase in pulse, tearing of the eyes, wrinkling of the forehead, or movement. Conversely, if the level of anesthesia is excessively deep, hypotension and bradycardia may occur. Unaltered, an extremely deep level of anesthesia may progress to cardiovascular and respiratory collapse. Maintenance of anesthesia requires a therapeutic balance between these levels to ensure patient safety and meet the needs of the surgeon.

As the surgery nears completion, anesthetic delivery is gradually decreased with the goal of the patient being capable of maintaining adequate spontaneous respiration by the end of the procedure and being responsive shortly thereafter. Depending on the anesthetic agents and ancillary drugs administered, such as nondepolarizing muscle relaxants, the use of specific reversal agents may be employed.

During the recovery phase, as the patient emerges from anesthesia, he or she passes through all stages in the reverse order. Since the classical stage of delirium (II) is not shortened on emergence, the inherent dangers of delirium are usually present whether a single agent or combination of agents was administered. In the stage of delirium, the patient may appear to be awake but does not respond to commands and may make random purposeless movements; to ensure safety, restraints should not be removed until the patient is about to be moved to the postoperative recovery area.

The greatest danger of stage II is hyperreflex sensitivity. Airway reflexes are increased, so the possibility of laryngospasm, which prevents ventilation, is increased. Stimulation of the airway, by oropharyngeal suctioning or extubation, must be avoided during this stage (Dershwitz, 1998). When the patient has safely emerged beyond the stage of delirium, the recovery phase begins.

Inhalation Anesthetic Agents

With the exception of nitrous oxide (N_2O), inhalation anesthetic agents are volatile liquids at room temperature. A calibrated vaporizer in the anesthesia machine vaporizes the liquid, which is then supplied to the patient via a carrier gas or gases. Oxygen (O_2) is always one of the carrier gases, but nitrous oxide may be added as a percentage of the total flow. This combination is traditionally charted as N_2O & O_2.

The percentage of oxygen delivered to the patient must always exceed the patient's metabolic oxygen requirements and be in greater concentration than the amount of oxygen found in room air. Most anesthesia machines have the capability of mixing room air with the oxygen flow for patients for whom 100% oxygen would be detrimental, such as those with chronic obstructive pulmonary disease or premature infants.

Most operating rooms have oxygen and nitrous oxide piped in from a central manifold outside the operating room suite. In some ambulatory surgical facilities, such as in physician offices and special procedure areas, oxygen and nitrous oxide must be supplied by portable tanks. By federal regulation, medical oxygen tanks are always colored green, and nitrous oxide tanks are blue.

Inhalation anesthetics may be used for induction and maintenance of anesthesia. Induction exclusively by inhalation is mainly used for small children and unique patient situations in which IV access is difficult to establish due to lack of patient cooperation or is extremely painful due to limited venous access.

Maintenance of general anesthesia is most commonly achieved with the use of an inhalation anesthetic because these agents allow more precise control of the anesthetic level (Eger, 2004). Uptake and distribution of the anesthetic is influenced by inspired anesthetic concentration, alveolar ventilation, fresh gas-flow rate from the anesthesia machine, blood/tissue solubility of the anesthetic, cardiac output, and functional residual capacity (FRC) of the lungs. Volatile anesthetic agents also produce varying degrees of skeletal muscle relaxation and may trigger malignant hyperthermia (MH) in genetically susceptible patients.

Potency of an inhalation anesthetic is related to its minimum alveolar concentration (MAC), the alveolar concentration of the gas at which 50% of individuals will not move in response to a skin incision. The greater the tissue solubility of an anesthetic, the lower its value for MAC; thus the least soluble volatile agent, desflurane, has a higher value for MAC than the most soluble, halothane (Eger, 2004).

Anesthesia providers often refer to the MAC of an anesthetic when referring to its potency. This should not be confused with the acronym sometimes used to designate monitored anesthesia care, which is also MAC. There is no relationship between the two terms.

Gaseous Agents

Nitrous Oxide

Nitrous oxide is the only inhalation anesthetic that is a gas at room temperature. Because it has the lowest blood solubility, it quickly produces its effect and is rapidly excreted in the exhaled breath, resulting in rapid awakening. The MAC of nitrous oxide is 110%, which is unattainable; therefore, it cannot be used as a complete anesthetic. To reach an adequate level of anesthesia, nitrous oxide must be combined with a volatile anesthetic, an IV agent, or both. Nitrous oxide increases the risk of postoperative nausea and vomiting but does not trigger malignant hyperthermia.

Volatile Agents

Isoflurane (Forane)

Isoflurane is widely used despite its pungent, irritating odor that may be overcome with the use of rapid-acting IV induction agents. Because it is primarily excreted unchanged by the lungs, uptake and elimination are rapid, and there is minimal chance of a cumulative effect from repeated exposure. The minimal amount of agent metabolized by the body is also a benefit for patients with severe systemic disease, but patients with severe hypovolemia may not tolerate its vasodilating effects well.

Although isoflurane increases heart rate, arrhythmias are much less common than with halothane. Isoflurane is less likely to sensitize the myocardium to the effects of catecholamines than other volatile anesthetics, making it more compatible with vasoconstrictor drugs used in conjunction with regional anesthetics. When used in low concentrations with oxygen, as an adjunct to local anesthesia, outpatients often meet discharge readiness criteria soon after the end of the procedure.

Desflurane (Suprane)

Desflurane is the least soluble of the volatile agents; therefore, it provides the most rapid onset of effect and the most rapid awakening. It is also the most irritating, so coughing and laryngospasm may result, causing problems during induction and emergence. Consequently, because of its pungent odor desflurane is avoided for induction.

Induction of anesthesia by inhalation is most commonly used for young children; however, the product label of desflurane warns against the agent's use for induction by mask in pediatric patients due to a high incidence of laryngospasm, coughing, breath holding, increase in secretions, and oxyhemoglobin desaturation (Eger, 2004).

In addition, if the concentration of desflurane is increased too quickly, hypertension and increased heart rate may occur before severe hypotension takes place. The desflurane product label advises against using the agent alone for induction for patients with coronary artery disease or if increases in heart rate or blood pressure are undesirable. Desflurane also causes an increase in salivation, so the use of an antisialagogue, such as atropine or glycopyrrolate, may be advisable.

Sevoflurane (Sevorane)

The most recently introduced volatile anesthetic in the United States has blood solubility slightly greater than desflurane but less than isoflurane. This rapid effect and recovery profile, together with a pleasant odor that does not cause airway irritation, make it appropriate for inhalation induction and a possible substitute for halothane (White & Recort-Freire, 2005).

Patients tend to be clearheaded on awakening, and sevoflurane does not sensitize the myocardium to the arrhythmic effects of epinephrine (Chung & Lam, 1997). Despite its high cost, the favorable pharmacologic properties of this inhalation anesthetic make it an increasingly popular choice for use in ambulatory settings.

Seizures have been reported, primarily in children and young adults, with sevoflurane. Desfluorane, isoflurane, halothane, and nitrous oxide do not cause seizures (Eger, 2004).

Sevoflurane was not approved in the United States until 1995 because of questions concerning its biodegradability. Although at the concentrations usually achieved, it is not thought to be associated with organ toxicity (Martin & Njoku, 2005), some clinicians prefer to avoid using sevoflurane with rebreathing techniques that put sevoflurane in contact with carbon dioxide absorption agents, such as Baralyme or Sodalime.

It is possible for absorbents to degrade potent inhalation anesthetics under certain circumstances, but unlike other agents sevoflurane can be degraded by moist or dry absorbents into compound A, which is believed to be nephrotoxic. Additionally, interaction with desiccated absorbents produces high temperature and carbon monoxide, potentially resulting in explosion or fire (Eger, 2004).

Halothane (Fluothane)

Halothane has a relatively sweet, pleasant odor; does not irritate the respiratory tract; and dilates the bronchi. These properties make it an excellent choice for induction without supplementation with an IV agent. As with other volatile agents, halothane causes dose-dependent hypotension; but unlike other volatile agents, it increases the sensitivity of the heart to the dysrhythmic effects of epinephrine. This effect is especially important in ambulatory surgery, where local anesthetics are commonly injected into the operative site to decrease general anesthesia requirements. Epinephrine should not be included in the local anesthetic mixture or serious arrhythmias may occur.

Halothane's major drawback is the occurrence of hepatic necrosis following repeated exposures.

Although rare, with a mechanism not completely understood, hepatic necrosis appears to occur most often with repeated use and in obese adults and children past puberty. Consequently, exposure is often minimized by changing to another inhalation anesthetic for maintenance after the induction benefits of halothane have been utilized (Morgan, Mikhail, & Murray, 2006). Because the newer volatile agent sevoflurane is, like halothane, not irritating to inhale, but unlike halothane does not cause hepatic toxicity, it appears to be replacing the use of halothane (White & Recart-Friere, 2005).

Desfluorane, isoflurane, and halothane are all metabolized to trifluoroacetate, which can cause hepatotoxicity through an immunologic response. However the incidence of hepatotoxicity depends on the amount of metabolism. Isoflurane and desflurane have much lower rates than halothane (Eger, 2004).

Intravenous Induction Agents

Rapid-acting IV hypnotic drugs are commonly used to induce anesthesia. Unconsciousness usually occurs within 15 to 30 seconds after IV injection, which is the time it takes for blood to circulate from the site of injection (e.g., arm) to the brain. Also referred to as IV anesthetic agents, these drugs produce a pleasant transition for the patient but have no analgesic affect. Without supplementation, IV hypnotic agents are only suitable for short surgical procedures with little associated pain because an unconscious patient may still react to painful stimuli. Doses sufficient to prevent response to pain may produce severe cardiovascular, respiratory, and central nervous system (CNS) depression. Consequently, these drugs are usually supplemented with nitrous oxide and oxygen, an opioid and nitrous oxide and oxygen, or a volatile inhalation agent and oxygen, depending on the requirements of the surgery.

Prior to induction, a small test dose of the hypnotic is usually administered to gauge patient response. This test dose is followed with a bolus dose sufficient to produce unconsciousness and the loss of the eyelash reflex. Because of their short duration of action, IV agent maintenance requires repeated incremental doses or continuous IV infusion. Table 3-2 summarizes IV anesthesia agents and supplemental drugs, including neuromuscular blocking agents.

Thiopental (Pentothal)

Thiopental is an ultra short-acting barbiturate widely used as an IV induction agent. Duration of action after a single induction dose is approximately 5 minutes, due to rapid redistribution from the brain to systemic tissue. It must then be metabolized, primarily by the liver. Only 1% is excreted unchanged in the urine. With repeated incremental doses, the duration of action becomes longer with each dose because of accumulation in peripheral tissues (Dershwitz, 1998). Consequently, thiopental produces a residual sedative effect characterized by grogginess and an inability to concentrate during

TABLE 3-2: INTRAVENOUS ANESTHESIA AGENTS AND SUPPLEMENTAL DRUGS

CLASSIFICATION	USE	EXAMPLES
Tranquilizers	Antianxiety, sedation	**Benzodiazepines:** midazolam (Versed), diazepam (Valium), lorazepam (Ativan) Specific reversal agent for benzodiazepines: flumazenil (Romazicon)
	Antiemetic, sedation	**Butyrophenone:** droperidol (Inapsine) **Phenothiazine:** promethazine (Phenergan)
Opioids	Analgesia, sedation	Fentanyl (Sublimaze), sufentanil (Sufenta), alfentanil (Alfenta), remifentanil (Ultiva), meperidine (Demerol), morphine sulfate, tramadol (Ultram). Specific opioid antagonist: naloxone (Narcan)
Agonist-antagonist Opioids	Analgesia, sedation	Butorphanol (Stadol), nalbuphine (Nubain) Generally produce less respiratory depression than pure opioid agonists such as fentanyl or morphine
Nonnarcotic, non-barbiturate hypnotic agents	Sedation, hypnosis, induction of anesthesia	Etomidate (Amidate), propofol (Diprivan), also used for maintenance of general anesthesia (total intravenous anesthesia) Sedation or unconsciousness induced in a dose-dependent fashion
Barbiturates	Sedation, hypnosis, induction of anesthesia	Thiopental (Pentothal), thiamylal (Surital), methohexital (Brevital)
Dissociative agent	Analgesia, induction of anesthesia	Ketamine (Ketalar) More often used in children; may be the sole anesthetic agent for some short procedures May be given intramuscularly
Neuromuscular blocking agents	Facilitation of intubation; provision of muscle relaxation for surgical procedure or for manipulation	**Depolarizing:** Succinylcholine (Quelicin, Anectine) **Nondepolarizing:** Pancuronium (Pavulon), atracurium (Tracrium), vecuronium (Norcuron), pipecuronium (Arduan), mivacurium (Mivacron), doxacurium (Nuromax), rocuronium (Zemuron), d-Tubocurarine (Curare), cisatracurium (Nimbex)

recovery. This pharmacokinetic profile makes thiopental unsuitable for continuous IV infusion, especially when rapid recovery is the objective (Chung & Lam, 1997; Dershwitz, 1998).

Large doses of thiopental may cause severe hypotension and depression of the myocardium in patients with congestive heart failure or hypovolemia. Patients taking beta-adrenergic antagonists or some antihypertensive medications may be unable to tolerate even small doses without adverse effects. Because thiopental is strongly alkaline, extravasation subcutaneously must be avoided; this is another reason for the use of a small test dose.

With insufficient depth of unconsciousness, manipulation of the airway, including any attempt to insert an oropharyngeal airway or aggressive positive-pressure ventilation, may provoke coughing, laryngospasm, or bronchospasm.

As with all barbiturates, thiopental may precipitate severe crisis or death in patients with acute intermittent porphyria or hereditary coproporphyria. It does not trigger MH. In addition, thiopental may be used to treat convulsions due to CNS toxic reactions, and it reduces intracranial pressure.

Methohexital (Brevital)

Methohexital is an ultra short-acting barbiturate, pharmacologically similar to thiopental. However, it is more potent and has a shorter duration of action. Methohexital's faster rate of hepatic clearance provides advantages for ambulatory surgery. There is less drowsiness during recovery and less cumulative effect with repeated dosage (Chung & Lam, 1997). Methohexital may be administered by continuous IV infusion for maintenance, which is followed by a relatively short recovery time.

Disadvantages of methohexital include coughing, hiccuping, and involuntary movement. Some discomfort may occur during injection, and methohexital's high alkalinity may cause tissue damage if extravasation occurs.

Propofol (Diprivan)

Propofol is the most recently introduced and most widely used IV sedative-hypnotic agent. Because of its rapid redistribution and elimination, propofol produces a faster recovery after an induction dose than other IV agents, making it a popular choice for ambulatory settings. This rapid recovery is characterized by clearheadedness and, in some patients, a sense of well-being. Psychomotor impairment also appears to be reduced, and there is a low incidence of nausea and vomiting; the drug may have an antiemetic effect.

Although not a barbiturate, propofol's hypnotic effect is, like that of thiopental, thought to be through action on the gamma-aminobutyric acid A receptor; however, propofol is suitable for continuous IV infusion. Patients are usually awake within 3 to 10 minutes after termination of an infusion regardless of duration or total dosage (Sweitzer, 1998). Propofol provides an alternative to barbiturates for patients with a history of allergic reaction to these drugs and patients with acute intermittent porphyria or hereditary coproporphyria.

Unlike thiopental, propofol does not increase airway irritability and may produce bronchodilation. An induction dose causes a greater decline in blood pressure and longer transient apnea than is seen with an equivalent dose of thiopental (Chung & Lam, 1997). Dosage and speed of administration should be reduced in elderly and debilitated patients (Tesniere & Servin, 2003).

A disadvantage of propofol is pain on injection. This pain may be lessened by using a larger vein, injecting lidocaine prior to the propofol, or adding lidocaine to the propofol solution. Involuntary movements or convulsions, especially in children, during induction have also been reported. When propofol is used as the sole maintenance agent, postoperative dysphoria may occur. However, the more usual and only partially understood elevation of mood seen on recovery from propofol contributes to the well-being and satisfaction of ambulatory patients (Tesniere & Servin, 2003).

Etomidate (Amidate)

Unlike other IV hypnotics, etomidate, an imidiazole derivative, has little depressant effect on the cardiovascular system and may be used as an induction agent for patients with hypovolemia and cardiac problems. It does not stimulate histamine release and is suitable for patients with asthma. Etomidate's onset and duration of action are similar to thiopental, but because of its rapid elimination, residual sedation and cumulative effect from repeated doses or continuous IV infusion are brief (Chung & Lam, 1997).

Etomidate may not be appropriate for ambulatory surgery because it has the highest incidence of postoperative nausea and vomiting of all the IV anesthetics. It may also cause considerable respiratory depression in conjunction with narcotics, especially if given by infusion (Kennedy, 1997). A single dose of etomidate may cause adrenocortical suppression for several hours, which may affect normal physiologic response to stress, such as surgery (Nagelhout & Boytim, 2001). The clinical significance of this effect in outpatients undergoing short procedures is controversial (Dershwitz, 1998).

Nursing Considerations

In the operating area, the patient should be the center of focus for the nurse, anesthesia provider, and surgeon. The following nursing actions apply to all anesthetized patients, and are especially relevant for the patient undergoing inhalation induction:

- While the patient is awake, avoid comments about equipment and staff that may be misinterpreted by the patient, especially after premedication may have produced an altered state of consciousness.
- Expose the patient as little as possible. Have warm blankets available to prevent hypothermia before induction, and to alleviate shivering should it occur during emergence.
- Maintain as quiet an atmosphere as possible, especially during induction and emergence.
- Once induction has begun, do not touch the patient without asking the anesthesia provider's permission, but stand by to assist in restraining the patient if it becomes necessary during an inhalation induction.
- Limit conversation about the patient during the procedure. Awareness during maintenance is rare, but keep in mind that hearing is the first sense to return.
- Assist in smoothly transferring the patient from the operating table to the stretcher.

Be prepared to assist the anesthesia provider immediately if asked. During the anesthetic process, seconds count.

- When steering the stretcher to the recovery area, do so as smoothly as possible to avoid inducing nausea and vomiting in susceptible individuals.

TOTAL INTRAVENOUS ANESTHESIA (TIVA)

The availability of rapid-acting IV sedative-hypnotics and opioid analgesics with fast onset and short duration have made it possible to induce and maintain anesthesia solely by the IV route. To maintain levels of unconsciousness appropriate to surgical stimulation, frequent small doses must be administered, gauged by signs of light anesthesia observed in the patient, to overcome the redistribution and elimination characteristics of these drugs. Continuous IV infusions are an alternative but also require adjustment depending on the stimulation of the surgery.

If the IV drugs used have cumulative or additive effects, delayed awakening may result. Because of its lack of cumulative effect, propofol is appropriate for continuous infusion, but it lacks analgesic properties and produces little amnesia. Propofol usually

Dysphoria = restlessness, agitation, exaggerated feelings

requires supplementation with a narcotic that has a rapid elimination profile. Midazolam may be used to provide amnesia. Awakening is typically rapid, but discharge may be delayed by persistent sedation, nausea, and pain (Conahan & Young, 1997).

Unlike inhalation anesthetics, the drugs used for TIVA provide no muscular relaxation. Depending on the requirements of the surgery, the administration of an NMBA may be necessary. When the patient is paralyzed by an NMBA, movement in response to painful stimulation, an important indicator of the patient's level of consciousness, is obscured. Signs such as tachycardia, tachypnea, elevated blood pressure, tearing, and wrinkling of the forehead become the primary indicators of response to pain and the need for additional medication.

A major disadvantage of TIVA is the increased possibility of patient awareness. Balanced anesthesia implies the use of combinations of drugs to produce the appropriate amount of analgesia, hypnosis, and muscular relaxation, but it also includes the use of low concentrations of an inhalation anesthetic. The possibility of patient awareness is reduced, but as with TIVA, the large amounts of IV narcotics that may be used with this technique tend to prolong cognitive recovery and increase the possibility of nausea and vomiting in ambulatory patients.

DISSOCIATIVE ANESTHESIA

Dissociative anesthesia, or neuroleptanesthesia, produces a mental state in which parts of the cerebrum are functionally dissociated. At subanesthetic levels, called neuroleptanalgesia, profound analgesia is accompanied by an appearance of wakefulness, yet there is a lack of communication. The patient's eyes may be open, but he or she is unaware of the surroundings.

Ketamine (Ketalar)

Ketamine is the only agent capable of producing anesthesia that may be administered IV or IM. After an IM injection, its duration of action is 15 to 20 minutes versus 5 to 10 minutes with IV injection. Because ketamine can be given IM, it can be used for uncooperative patients, especially children, and when IV accessibility is limited or would be unusually painful. For these reasons, ketamine is frequently used for burn patients, pediatric diagnostic procedures, and gravely ill patients.

Under ketamine anesthesia, the patient is usually able to maintain his or her airway and retains laryngeal reflexes; however, airway obstruction or aspiration still may occur. Increased salivation and mucus production may require the use of an antisialagogue, such as atropine or glycopyrrolate. Ketamine also dilates the bronchi.

The use of ketamine for ambulatory surgery may be questionable because of the bad dreams and dysphoria that patients often experience during recovery. Midazolam and a quiet atmosphere may reduce unpleasant emergence reactions. However, ketamine's unique ability to support the cardiovascular system and its ability to be administered IM, make it useful in emergency, accident, and disaster situations outside a hospital setting. Because it increases intracranial pressure, ketamine should be avoided when head injury is suspected.

NEUROMUSCULAR BLOCKING AGENTS

To relax skeletal muscle during anesthesia, an NMBA, or muscle relaxant, may be required to allow adequate surgical exposure, as in abdominal surgery; permit joint manipulation during orthopedic surgery; and decrease the insufflation pressure required for laparoscopic procedures (Dershwitz, 1998). Muscle relaxants are also used to facilitate the insertion of an endotracheal tube by relaxing the vocal cords, which reduces the risk of injury.

Neuromuscular blockade occurs primarily at the neuromuscular junction (NMJ) at the cholinergic-nicotinic receptors on the motor endplate. Muscle relaxants cause paralysis of striated muscle, but they do not affect awareness, cognition, or pain perception. It is essential that the patient be unconscious before receiving an NMBA and that respiration be supported until paralysis has worn off or been pharmacologically reversed.

The mode of action of NMBAs is either depolarizing or nondepolarizing.

Depolarizing NMBAs

Succinylcholine (Anectine, Quelicin) is the only depolarizing muscle relaxant in widespread clinical use. When molecules of succinylcholine occupy receptors on the motor endplate, the muscle transiently contracts, causing fasciculations. But as depolarization persists, neuromuscular transmission is interrupted, and the muscle becomes flaccid (Kervin, 2002). Succinylcholine produces muscular relaxation in less than 1 minute, and a single dose lasts approximately 3 to 5 minutes.

This rapid onset and short duration of action make it well-suited for ambulatory surgery, as well as relatively short procedures in general. For the same reasons, succinylcholine is usually administered by continuous infusion. The initial muscle fasciculation, although often not observable, may be responsible for postoperative muscle pain. Generalized muscular aches seem to occur more frequently in outpatients, especially young adults, after minor surgery.

Although there is wide personal variance due to disease or genetics, a large total dosage of succinylcholine or prolonged duration of administration may result in a persistent phase I depolarizing block, or the production of a phase II block that mimics nondepolarizing blockade. At present, there is no antagonist or reversal agent clinically available for succinylcholine's phase I blockade. However, a phase II blockade may, in some instances, respond to reversal agents used for nondepolarizing muscle relaxants (Morgan, Mikhail, & Murray, 2006).

Because succinylcholine is metabolized by the enzyme pseudocholinesterase (plasma cholinesterase), reduced levels of this enzyme may prolong its effect. Causes of reduced plasma cholinesterase include liver disease, malignancy, chemotherapeutic medications, and pregnancy. Echothiophate eyedrops, used in the treatment of glaucoma, and neostigmine are contraindications to the use of succinylcholine. Genetic abnormalities that produce atypical plasma cholinesterase may significantly prolong the effect of succinylcholine.

Succinylcholine may trigger MH in genetically susceptible patients. Its use in children is controversial because a child may have a genetically determined myopathy that is associated with MH but has not yet become symptomatic (Dershwitz, 1998).

Nondepolarizing NMBAs

Stimulatory motor nerve impulses cause acetylcholine to be released at the NMJ. Nondepolarizing muscle relaxants prevent acetylcholine from binding to its receptors to cause muscle contraction. They require 2 to 3 minutes to achieve full effect, which may last 45 minutes or longer, depending on the particular relaxant. However, nondepolarizing muscle relaxants may be pharmacologically reversed with the use of a cholinesterase inhibitor such as neostigmine, pyridostigmine, or edrophonium (Tensilon). Atropine or glycopyrrolate (Robinul) are usually administered along with the reversal agent to offset undesirable parasympathetic effects, most commonly bradycardia and increased respiratory secretions.

Short-acting nondepolarizing agents, such as mivacurium (Mivacron), with a duration of 15 minutes, and intermediate-acting agents, vecuronium (Norcuron), atracurium (Tracrium), and rocuronium (Zemuron), and cisatracurium (Nimbex) are suitable for ambulatory surgical procedures. These drugs do not trigger MH but may cause hypotension due to histamine release. Cisatracurim, however, does not cause histamine release.

The effect of nondepolarizing muscle relaxants may be potentiated by commonly used medications such as certain antibiotics, lidocaine, quinidine, beta-antagonists, and calcium channel blockers such as verapamil. Mivacurium, the shortest acting depolarizing NMBA, may be prolonged by inadequate levels of plasma cholinesterase.

Peripheral Nerve Stimulation

By delivering a strong electrical stimulus to a peripheral nerve and observing the pattern and strength of muscle twitch that occurs, the amount of existing neuromuscular blockade can be assessed. This technique may be used during or at the completion of surgery and is frequently used to test the patient's recovery of muscle strength. If accessible, the ulnar nerve in the forearm is usually the nerve tested.

Electric nerve stimulation may be applied in the form of tetany, train of four (TOF), double burst, or single twitch, all of which require skilled interpretation. TOF is probably the most easily interpreted for the postanesthesia care nurse (Kervin, 2002). However, the level of electric current necessary may be painful for the recovering patient and may also irritate the skin at the site being used. (Kervin, 2002; Viby-Mogenson, 2005).

Physical assessment of residual neuromuscular blockade is readily discernible in the recovering patient by asking the patient for a tight hand grip or to extend the tongue. The most reliable indication of adequate muscular strength may be the patient's ability to hold the head off the bed for 5 seconds (Kervin, 2002).

Peripheral nerve stimulation can also be used to differentiate the type of blockade present; normally, depolarizing and nondepolarizing muscle relaxants produce different patterns of response. However, if a phase II block has occurred subsequent to depolarizing blockade, the response resembles that of nondepolarizing blockade, and is indicative of the untoward occurrence. This technique may also be used diagnostically to determine if apnea is due to central respiratory depression rather than muscular paralysis (Chung & Lam, 1997).

Additionally, in a lightly sedated patient who is able to interact with the anesthesia provider an electrical nerve stimulator may be used to precisely locate the nerve to be blocked so the local anesthetic may be injected closely without actually touching the nerve (McCamant, 2006).

REGIONAL ANESTHESIA

As the name implies, regional anesthesia techniques produce loss of sensation in a particular area of the body. This effect is accomplished with the injection of drugs, collectively referred to as local anesthetics, that can temporarily interrupt, or block, the conduction of impulses along nerve fibers. Consequently, these techniques are often referred to as conduction anesthesia or simply as "blocks." By altering the nerve membrane's permeability to sodium (Na), local anesthetic agents impede the propagation of the nerve impulse. Nerve diameter, myelination, and conduction velocity of the nerve fibers all affect this progression.

Analgesia and motor impairment develop in the anesthetized area while the patient remains conscious and in full control of his or her airway. The order of loss of nerve function is: pain, temperature, touch, proprioception, and skeletal muscle tone (Drug Consult, 2006). When used as the sole anesthetic technique, regional anesthesia causes little systemic physiologic alteration. However, in addition to sensory and motor fibers, sympathetic nerves are affected, causing peripheral vasodilation and erythema due to unopposed parasympathetic effect (McCamant, 2006). A benefit of local anesthetics is their anti-inflammatory action that is most likely due to modulation of neutrophil function (White & Durieux, 2005).

By using a local anesthetic with a duration of effect appropriate to the anticipated length of the surgical procedure, the ambulatory surgical patient may be expected to be quickly recovered and ready for discharge. However, the use of premedication or intraoperative sedation may considerably affect home readiness; psychomotor function may be impaired for several hours after surgery when such medications are necessary. A poorly selected candidate for regional anesthesia, who requires heavy sedation, may negate the fast recovery benefits.

Although it is generally accepted that regional anesthesia alone does not affect postoperative psychomotor performance, studies show that with high doses of lidocaine (Xylocaine), psychomotor performance may be impaired for 1 to 1.5 hours. This impairment has not been demonstrated with mepivacaine (Carbocaine) or lidocaine with epinephrine. Long-acting local anesthetics, such as bupivacaine (Marcaine) or etidocaine (Duranest), may also impair psychomotor performance for at least 2 hours. When no contraindications exist, the use of short-acting local anesthetics with epinephrine may be preferable for ambulatory surgical procedures.

Regional anesthesia is not a panacea for any class of physical status or any type of surgery. Contraindications for regional anesthesia include:

- *Extremes of age and mental status* – inability of the patient to cooperate.
- *Coagulopathy or anticoagulation therapy* – potential for bleeding causing compression of the nerves or tissue damage.
- *Infection at the site of injection* – spread of infection via the needle and decreased effectiveness of the local anesthetic agent in the acidic tissues near an infection.
- *Patient preference* – patient's refusal of regional anesthesia because of apprehension about what they will see and hear in the operating room or fear of paralysis.
- *Preexisting neurologic deficits* – relative contraindications that must be evaluated on a case-by-case basis.
- *Systemic disease* – hepatic or renal impairment that may alter metabolism of local anesthetics, increasing the risk of systemic toxicity. Patients with coronary artery disease may respond adversely to the effects of epinephrine mixed with the anesthetic.

In an ambulatory surgical setting, a potential disadvantage of regional anesthesia is the time required to perform the block and the delayed onset of anesthetic effect. This disadvantage may be overcome by performing the block in a designated area outside the operating room. Full resuscitation equipment should be immediately available in the area where regional anesthesia is performed, including medications used to treat local anesthetic toxicity.

Consent for regional anesthesia must also be obtained before the administration of any sedation or injection of any local anesthetics. Policies for obtaining informed consent vary with the facility, but both types of anesthesia (general and regional) should be addressed. A signed consent form is not necessarily legal evidence of consent if the patient does not understand the exact terms of the agreement (Darwin Professional Underwriters, Inc., 2006).

Similarly, patients scheduled for regional anesthesia must be prepared preoperatively as done for general anesthesia. Maintaining NPO status is a precaution in the event of an adverse drug reaction or the need for general anesthesia. However, this protocol is becoming less common and depends largely on the type of procedure scheduled. Preexisting neurologic deficits, discovered from the history or preoperative examination, should be documented to prevent misdiagnosis of possible postanesthetic neurologic problems (Gaiser, 1997).

Mild anxiolytic premedication may improve the patient's anesthetic experience and increase safety. Nerve injury may be reduced because non-apprehensive patients are less likely to move during injection of the local anesthetic. In addition, large total doses of local anesthetic are less likely to cause CNS toxicity if a benzodiazepine is given preoperatively to raise the seizure threshold.

For the very anxious ambulatory surgical patient, premedication may best be accomplished with the use of small IV doses given just prior to the placement of the block. Because there is some degree of discomfort associated with most regional blocks, a small dose of a short-acting opioid, such as alfentanil, may be indicated to produce a brief period of intense analgesia (Morgan, Mikhail, & Murray, 2006).

Monitoring during regional anesthesia focuses on detecting delayed local anesthetic toxicity from excessive tissue absorption (typically 15 to 60 minutes after injection), ensuring adequate ventilation and oxygenation, and managing the consequences of surgical stress, such as tourniquet pain or blood loss. Patients with adequate blocks may be sedated, and the use of supplemental oxygen is appropriate (d'Amours, 1997). Maintaining IV access is advisable during all types of regional anesthesia.

Spinal Anesthesia

Also referred to as subarachnoid anesthesia or intrathecal anesthesia, spinal anesthesia is produced by injecting an appropriate local anesthetic into the cerebrospinal fluid (CSF) that bathes and cushions the spinal cord and spinal nerve roots. CSF circulates in the subarachnoid space between the arachnoid membrane and the pia mater membrane, which closely covers the spinal cord. In the adult, the spinal cord extends only to the second lumbar vertebra (L2), whereas the subarachnoid space extends to the second sacral vertebra (S2), within the dural sac. Using strict sterile technique, the local anesthetic is injected well below the L2 level to avoid contact with the spinal cord. Patients tend to fear spinal anesthesia because they wrongly believe the anesthetic is injected into the spinal cord.

Onset of anesthesia is rapid, occurring within minutes. Depending on the baricity, or specific gravity of the local anesthetic compared to that of CSF, the anesthetic moves either cephalad (i.e., upward), caudad (i.e., downward), or remains near the site of injection. Consequently, the position of the patient is extremely important in controlling the level of anesthesia. The position of the operating table should be adjusted only by the anesthesia provider. It takes 10 to 20 minutes for the anesthesia level to become reasonably stable after injection. Hyperbaric (heavier than CSF) anesthetic solutions, which will move downward by gravity in the subarachnoid space, are most frequently used; therefore, the patient's head must be constantly supported by a firm pillow, and the Trendelenburg position must be avoided.

The level of spinal anesthesia using a hyperbaric solution is also affected by the dose of local anesthetic; total volume injected; speed of injection; coughing or straining by the patient after injection; and increased intra-abdominal pressure, as with pregnancy and obesity. Sensory level of anesthesia is usually judged by pinprick testing to determine the dermatome, or skin region supplied by a particular spinal nerve, level of sensation. Sympathetic blockade extends above the dermatome level of sensory loss. If the level of anesthesia ascends to the upper thoracic or cervical levels, respiratory paralysis may occur.

Autonomic (sympathetic and parasympathetic) fibers are the first to be anesthetized, followed by the nerve fibers affecting touch, pain, motor control, and proprioception. Because recovery occurs in the reverse order, a patient may be able to stand and move, yet may experience orthostatic hypotension due to incomplete autonomic recovery. Motor control is lost first in the toes and moves upward.

The profound sympathetic blockade often results in hypotension, which may be severe in pregnant and geriatric patients and may be accompanied by nausea and retching. Mild hypotension may respond to oxygen administration and, except in patients at risk for congestive heart failure, temporary increase in the flow of IV fluids. If hypotension is severe, vasopressors may be required. Oxygen supplementation is appropriate during the course of spinal anesthesia, especially for patients who have been sedated.

Profound hypotension and bradycardia with loss of consciousness and apnea indicate that total spinal anesthesia has occurred. Along with circulatory support, tracheal intubation and controlled ventilation with 100% oxygen is necessary. Recovery may be complete if action is taken promptly (Chung & Lam, 1997).

Absolute and relative contraindications to spinal anesthesia exist (Brown, D.L., 2005; Kleinman & Mikhail, 2006).

- Absolute contraindications to spinal anesthesia include:
  - lack of patient consent
  - infection at the site of needle insertion
  - coagulopathy or anticoagulation therapy
  - uncontrolled shock or hypovolemia
  - increased intracranial pressure
  - severe aortic or mitral stenosis.
- Relative contraindications to spinal anesthesia include:
  - bacteremia
  - herniation of an intervertebral disk
  - previous back surgery
  - neurologic disease
  - psychosis or dementia
  - surgery of uncertain duration.

Spinal Anesthesia for Ambulatory Surgery

Spinal anesthesia may be suitable for ambulatory surgical procedures involving the lower half of the body; however, discharge may be delayed due to persistent orthostatic hypotension, prolonged motor or sensory blockade, or urinary retention. Males are more likely to experience delayed return of bladder tone resulting in urinary retention (White & Recart-Friere, 2005) and persistent inability to void may require hospital admission (Long, 1997).

In an outpatient setting, it is important that the local anesthetic used for spinal anesthesia has a duration of effect appropriate to the anticipated duration of the surgical procedure to ensure rapid recovery and discharge. Consequently, short-acting agents are preferable whenever possible. Lidocaine for shorter procedures and bupivacaine for longer procedures have been the most commonly used for ambulatory surgical patients, and are discussed under "Local Anesthetic Agents."

Postdural Puncture Headache

A possible postoperative complication of spinal anesthesia, postdural puncture headache (PDPH) appears to occur more frequently in outpatients. Incidence may be as high as 18% in ambulatory surgical patients (Conahan & Young, 1997). Younger patients appear to be at greater risk. Preoperative informed consent should include a discussion of the risk of PDPH and treatment options (Long, 1997).

PDPH is thought to result from leakage of CSF from the subarachnoid space through the dura mater. This leakage allows the brain and its supporting structures to sag, causing traction on pain-sensitive vascular structures (Morgan, Mikhail, & Murray, 2006). Size and design of the spinal needle are believed to be contributing factors to PDPH. For ambulatory patients, the use of the more expensive pencil-point style spinal needle may be advisable.

PDPH usually takes 24 to 72 hours to develop and is aggravated by sitting and standing. Treatment includes lying flat in bed, analgesics, and liberal fluid intake. In protracted cases, an autologous "blood patch" is usually effective. This intervention involves injecting 10 to 15 ml of the patient's own blood into the epidural space at the level of the original lumbar puncture to seal the dural leak (Chung & Lam, 1997). Autologous epidural blood patches relieve PDPH in 90% of cases (Brown, D.L., 2005).

Epidural Anesthesia

The outermost membrane that encircles the spinal cord is the dura mater. The epidural space is outside the dura mater. Local anesthetics injected into this space can block neural transmission by anesthetizing spinal nerve roots, blocking spinal nerves as they emerge from the intervertebral foramina, and diffusing intrathecally (Chung & Lam, 1997).

Epidural anesthesia may be an alternative to spinal anesthesia, but a dose approximately 10 times larger than that used for spinal anesthesia is required to obtain a comparable level. Anesthesia develops segmentally, and maximum effect occurs in 10 to 15 minutes. Because it is injected into a space, rather than fluid, spread of the local anesthetic is not closely dependent on the patient's position.

For better control of dosage and to allow repeated administration for long procedures, a catheter can be threaded into the epidural space. The catheter should be clearly labeled, and nothing should be injected into it by anyone other than the anesthesia provider. Once established, epidural anesthesia is suitable for intra-abdominal, perineal, and lower extremity surgery. Epidural anesthesia is widely used for the pain of childbirth.

As with spinal anesthesia, hypotension is a potential complication, but, like sensory loss, may occur more gradually. PDPH does not occur unless there is inadvertent puncture of the dura mater. Because of the larger needle used, PDPH, should it occur, may be worse. Epidural hematoma and accidental total spinal anesthesia are uncommon but potential complications. Contraindications to epidural anesthesia are similar to those for spinal anesthesia.

Peripheral Nerve Blocks

A peripheral nerve block may involve a single nerve or a plexus of nerves. To avoid neuropathy, the local anesthetic is injected adjacent to the nerve or nerves to be anesthetized, where it diffuses into the neural tissue. Anesthesia develops in the area of distribution of the blocked nerve. Profound analgesia is possible, although the amount of motor paralysis depends on the concentration achieved. Proprioception may not be affected, and the patient may still be aware of a limb being positioned or skin being prepared for surgery.

Sufficient time is needed for diffusion of the local anesthetic through connective tissue barriers surrounding the nerves, so repeatedly testing the area before reasonable time has passed for the effect to occur may cause the patient to become anxious. Loss of response to a pinprick and decreased sensitivity to cold indicate the onset of anesthesia. Before incision, the surgeon should retest the site, for example by gently probing it with a scalpel or clamp, to confirm the adequacy of the block (d'Amours, 1997).

Brachial Plexus Block

Nerves in the brachial plexus supply virtually all of the sensory and motor innervation of the arm. There are three possible injection approaches: interscalene, supraclavicular, and axillary.

The interscalene approach is suitable for shoulder and upper arm surgery, but there is a danger of inadvertent injection into the cervical subarachnoid or epidural spaces, resulting in spinal or epidural anesthesia. Inadvertent injection of the local anesthetic into the vertebral artery may result in systemic toxicity. Phrenic nerve block and neuropathy of the C6 nerve root are also potential complications associated with this technique.

Supraclavicular injection, as well as infraclavicular injection, produces anesthesia of the elbow, wrist, and hand. With these approaches there is a risk of inadvertent puncture of the pleura, resulting in pneumothorax. If the patient coughs as the needle is being advanced or complains of respiratory distress, oxygen should be administered by mask immediately and appropriate treatment instituted. These patients should be monitored for dyspnea or absent breath sounds (McCamant, 2006).

The axillary approach is suitable for surgery of the hand and forearm. There is no risk of pneumothorax, but a large dose of local anesthetic is required, increasing the risk of systemic toxicity. Additionally, the arm must be able to be raised to allow access to the axilla. Ipsilateral phrenic nerve paralysis and ophthalmic changes may be associated with brachial plexis block, but treatment may not be necessary unless the patient is annoyed by the symptoms (Wedel & Horlacker, 2005)

For ambulatory surgery, a brachial plexus block provides the benefit of postoperative analgesia. However, because of the resulting prolonged lack of sensation and impaired mobility, there is a danger of accidental injury to the arm after discharge of an ambulatory patient.

Ilioinguinal-Iliohypogastric Block

Blockade of the ilioinguinal and iliohypogastric nerves provides anesthesia suitable for inguinal herniorrhaphy, orchiectomy, and orchidopexy. Because the autonomic nervous system is not blocked, sympathetically mediated pain and parasympathetically mediated nausea and vomiting may occur during traction on the peritoneum (Morgan, Mikhail, & Murray, 2006). Analgesia extends well into the postoperative period, especially when coupled with inguinal field infiltration. Such infiltration, or block, is produced by injecting a relatively large volume of local anesthetic in the general location of nerves supplying the region to be anesthetized (Tetzlaff, 1996).

Long-acting local anesthetics are often selected with the anticipated benefit of postoperative analgesia, but when long-acting agents are used for ilioinguinal or iliohypogastric nerve blocks, the anesthetic solution may spread to the femoral nerve, resulting in quadriceps weakness and short-term postoperative difficulty in walking. For the outpatient, femoral nerve involvement may be avoided by using a more dilute solution, although the onset of the block might be less rapid. When used in conjunction with general anesthesia for pediatric outpatients, infiltrating only the wound may be preferable (Zwass, 2005). Similarly, femoral or sciatic nerve blocks for surgery on the lower extremities may not be appropriate for outpatients who must be able to walk in order to meet discharge criteria.

Local Infiltration and Topical Application

One of the most commonly used local anesthesia techniques for ambulatory surgical procedures, local infiltration involves the injection of a local anesthetic into the skin and subcutaneous tissue in the area of the operative site, blocking transmission at the nerve endings where pain impulses would arise. Topical application produces analgesia and anesthesia over a limited surface area and is most frequently used for mucous membranes, where it is rapidly absorbed. Cocaine may be used topically for some nasal, upper respiratory or ophthalmic procedures, which makes careful monitoring of the patient for hypertension, dysrhythmias, or seizures essential.

Preemptive Analgesia

The principle of preemptive analgesia is that therapeutic intervention is instituted before pain occurs rather than in response to pain. Studies have shown that infiltration of a local anesthetic into the operative area before the incision is made prevents the usual neural response to tissue injury. The anesthetized peripheral nerve endings are incapable of transmitting the pain impulse to the dorsal horns of the spinal cord where it would then be conveyed to the brain and interpreted as pain.

Referred to as the gate-control theory, the gateway for painful stimuli transmitted by small-diameter nerve fibers is opened when the incision is made. By stopping pain perception at its source, the transmission to the brain is minimal to none (Roberge & McEwen, 1998).

General anesthesia obtunds the brain's memory of surgical pain but does not stop the spinal cord from reacting to the stimulus. When no longer anesthetized, the brain receives the stimulus from the spinal cord and interprets it as pain. However, if a local anesthetic has been injected into the operative site, the intensity of postoperative pain may be significantly reduced.

Infiltration of a local anesthetic into the wound during surgery or at closure also reduces postoperative need for strong analgesics, but less effectively than infiltration before the nerve endings have been injured when the incision is made. Postoperative pain is minimized and delayed, at least for the duration of the local anesthetic's effect, which in the case of long-acting agents such as bupivacaine, may be for 6 hours or more. Preemptive analgesia may effectively reduce the need for narcotic analgesia during the first several days of surgery (Connor & Fogg, 1999).

Surgeons may be encouraged to use this technique if the nurse asks what type and strength of local injection he or she wishes, rather than asking whether a local anesthetic injection will be used (Conner & Fogg, 1999). The use of local wound infiltration should be encouraged more frequently for all surgical patients, particularly in the outpatient setting (Mulroy & Owens, 1997).

IV Perfusion Block

This regional technique, also known as a Bier block, is especially useful in ambulatory settings for surgical procedures of short duration on the forearm, hand, and foot. Advantages include rapid onset, rapid recovery and discharge, and high reliability. The technique involves occluding the circulation of the arm or foot using a pneumatic tourniquet above the operative site. Due to the time limitation for interruption of circulation by an occluding tourniquet, procedures of 45 minutes or less are most suitable, with 90 minutes considered the maximum duration for safety (Wedel & Horlacher, 2005).

The extremity is elevated and, starting at the fingers, tightly wrapped with an Esmarch elastic bandage to exsanguinate it. The tourniquet is then inflated, and local anesthetic is injected IV to distend the veins. The tourniquet prevents the exit of the local anesthetic from the extremity as the anesthetic diffuses out of the veins to block small nerves and nerve endings.

Once the anesthetic is injected, the tourniquet must remain inflated 15 to 20 minutes, regardless of a shorter duration of surgery, to reduce the risk of systemic toxicity when the local anesthetic is released into the bloodstream. After surgery, the tourniquet is slowly, or intermittently, deflated, and any remaining anesthetic is gradually released into the systemic circulation. Sensation usually returns within 2 to 5 minutes.

Pain at the tourniquet site may become intense. This pain may be alleviated by using a double tourniquet where the upper section is first inflated for the IV injection. When discomfort develops around the tourniquet, the lower, or distal, section is inflated in the area that has become anesthetized, and the upper section is released. Failure of the tourniquet or inadvertent release before 15 minutes may result in seizures or cardiovascular collapse caused by the rapid distribution of a large dose of local anesthetic into the bloodstream.

In some instances, the rapid return of sensation may be considered a disadvantage for ambulatory patients because there is a lack of postoperative analgesia. In addition, the exsanguination process may be too uncomfortable for patients with a painful extremity.

Local Anesthetic Agents

Local anesthetics differ in potency, onset of action, duration of effect, and potency (see Table 3-3). There are two main pharmacologic classes, or types, of local anesthetics, amides and esters. Amides are detoxified by the liver, and esters are metabolized by ester hydrolysis and plasma cholinesterase (pseudocholinesterase). Patients with liver impairment or decreased plasma cholinesterase levels may have a prolonged local anesthetic effect. Because most local anesthetics and their metabolites are excreted by the kidneys, adequate renal function is also a consideration (Drug Consult, 2006).

The range of properties of various anesthetic agents offers flexible clinical usages; lidocaine and bupivacaine have been popular choices. However, after many years of clinical use, adverse properties of both agents were identified and studied. The cardiac side effects possible with bupivacaine were resolved by adjusting the concentrations used (White & Durieux, 2005). Additionally, ropivacaine, with similar anesthetic properities but without potential cardiotoxic effect was introduced.

Similarly, the prototypical local anesthetic lidocaine was found to be capable of causing transient neuropathies, such as radicular nerve root irritation and more rarely cauda equine syndrome. Although transient neurologic symptoms have been documented as possible with every local anesthetic used for spinal anesthesia, they appear to occur more frequently with the use of lidocaine. This trend is especially apparent when lidocaine is used for ambulatory procedures for knee arthroscopy or gynecological surgeries that require the lithotomy position (Mulroy, 2006). Whether altering the dose or concentration of lidocaine reduces the possibility of these effects occurring is controversial (Brown, D.L., 2005; White & Durieux, 2005).

All local anesthetics, regardless of the type, are capable of producing systemic toxic reactions. Systemic toxicity results when there is a high blood concentration of local anesthetic, which may be due to rapid absorption of a nontoxic dose, inadvertent injection of anesthetic into a blood vessel, or administration of a toxic dose (Chung & Lam, 1997). Peak blood concentrations may be delayed for 15 to 60 minutes after injection, so patients must be continuously monitored.

Symptoms of developing CNS toxicity include:

- light-headedness
- tinnitus
- metallic taste in the mouth
- vision disturbances
- numbness around the mouth
- vague sensations not easily defined by the patient
- agitation
- muscle twitches
- uncontrollable shaking.

TABLE 3-3: PROPERTIES OF LOCAL ANESTHETICS

Generic Name	Trade Name	Type	Onset	Duration	Potency	Toxicity
Procaine	Novocain	Ester	Rapid	Short	Low	Low
Lidocaine	Xylocaine	Amide	Rapid	Moderate	Moderate	Moderate
Chloroprocaine	Nesacaine	Ester	Rapid	Short	Low	Low
Mepivacaine	Carbocaine	Amide	Moderate	Moderate	Moderate	Moderate
Bupivacaine	Marcaine	Amide	Slow	Very long	High	High
Tetracaine	Pontocaine	Ester	Slow	Long	High	High
Ropivacaine	Naropin	Amide	Slow	Long	High	Moderate

If CNS toxicity is untreated, seizures (convulsions), unconsciousness, and coma may ensue. Benzodiazepines given for preoperative sedation or procedural sedation elevate the seizure threshold and may provide some prophylaxis (Morgan, Mikhail, & Murray, 2006). IV diazepam is the drug of choice in the treatment of CNS toxicity (Chung & Lam, 1997). Thiopental is effective in treating convulsions, but an anesthetic dose may be required.

Seizures increase oxygen requirements while reducing adequate respiration. Oxygen must be administered effectively to avoid hypoxia. If unconsciousness or coma occur, endotracheal intubation may be required to support ventilation.

Cardiovascular toxicity is characterized by:

- hypotension
- bradycardia
- dysrhythmia.

If cardiovascular toxicity is undetected or untreated, circulatory collapse and cardiac arrest may occur. Immediate treatment includes oxygen administration, IV fluids for intravascular expansion, and pharmacologic cardiac support.

Patients receiving regional anesthesia without premedication may exhibit symptoms that must be differentiated from those of toxicity. The anxious or frightened patient may appear agitated and suffer from nausea and vomiting. A vasovagal response may be accompanied by hypotension, bradycardia, and faintness. Administering oxygen and increasing IV fluid flow rate, if not contraindicated, are advisable while the evaluation is being made.

For peripheral nerve blocks and infiltration, larger volumes produce better blockade, so less concentrated solutions of local anesthetic are used to prevent overdosage and possible toxicity. Moderate concentrations, such as 1% to 1.5% lidocaine or 0.50% bupivacaine, are used commonly for nerve blocks, whereas dilute solutions, such as 0.50% lidocaine or 0.125% bupivacaine, are used for infiltration when large volumes are necessary (d'Amours, 1997).

Vasoconstrictors

Vasoconstrictors added to local anesthetics slow tissue absorption, which prolongs the duration of anesthesia and reduces toxicity. Epinephrine is most frequently used in oncentrations of 1:100,000 or less. Using lidocaine, peripheral nerve blocks last for 60 to 90 minutes; adding epinephrine may extend these times by 50%. With bupivacaine, blocks may last more than 3 hours; with epinephrine added, blocks may last for more than 12 hours.

Vasoconstrictors should not be used for blocks in which distal circulation may be compromised by vasoconstriction, such as digital blocks for fingers or toes (d'Amours, 1997). They must be used with caution in elderly patients and are contraindicated for patients with unstable angina, patients with cardiac dysrhythmias, hyperthyroid patients, and patients with uteroplacental insufficiency (Kost, 2004).

Epinephrine added to local anesthetic solutions to delay absorption and prolong the anesthetic effect may cause tachycardia, diaphoresis, pallor, anxiety, changes in mental perception, and strange subjective feelings for the patient that may be misinterpreted as an allergic reaction.

Allergic Reactions

Hypersensitivity, or allergic reactions to local anesthetics, such as urticaria, bronchospasms, and anaphylaxis, have been reported but are rare. They may be more associated with the ester-type anesthetics because these drugs are metabolized to para-aminobenzoic acid (PABA), which is known to cause allergic reactions under other circumstances. However, bacteriostatic and preservative additives may be responsible for some of the reported reactions.

Careful questioning of the patient as part of the preoperative assessment is important. A patient who relates urticaria and difficulty breathing during a previous anesthetic probably had an allergic reaction, whereas a patient who describes palpitations and a headache immediately after injection of the local anesthetic probably had effects from the epinephrine in the local anesthetic solution, which may have been injected intravascularly (Vitkun, 1997).

Nursing Considerations

When the regional anesthetic administration does not require the participation of an anesthesia provider, monitoring of the patient usually becomes the responsibility of the perioperative nurse. Periorbital and retrobulbar blocks are examples of peripheral nerve blocks extensively used in ambulatory surgical settings for cataract extraction and lens implantations, which may be performed by the operating ophthalmologist. In addition to checking and recording the blood pressure and vital signs every 15 minutes, the nurse should be thoroughly familiar with the pharmacologic profiles of local anesthetics, supportive treatment for toxic reactions, and the location and use of emergency medications and equipment.

Monitoring and supportive treatment should be carried out according to the established policies of the facility and documented on the patient's medical record. The Association of PeriOperative Registered Nurses (AORN) recommends that documentation of monitoring of the patient receiving local anesthesia should provide evidence of continuous assessment.

Fundamental patient monitoring parameters include respiration, blood pressure, pulse, oxygenation, and signs of adverse reactions. Monitoring involves comprehensive vigilant care that protects the patient from harm. For example, any change in the patient's position necessitates reevaluation of possible pressure points and padding to prevent injury, and IV fluids must be monitored for possible extravasation. Additionally, the nurse should act as an intermediary between the patient and surgeon by keeping the surgeon advised of any changes in the patient's condition and providing emotional support through direct communication with the patient. Patient monitoring is discussed further in Chapter 4.

Understanding the concepts and techniques of regional anesthesia prepares the nurse to appropriately attend to the patient's anxieties and needs preoperatively, intraoperatively, and postoperatively. The knowledgeable nurse may help relieve the following common patient concerns about regional anesthesia.

- Fear of feeling pain during the procedure
- Fear that the anesthesia will wear off before the surgery is completed
- Fear of paralysis due to the local anesthetic

By reinforcing, and perhaps further defining, information provided by the anesthesia provider or surgeon, the nurse may facilitate patient acceptance and relieve his or her anxiety.

In addition, keeping the product information sheet or package insert from all regularly used local anesthetics readily available in the operating room provides an excellent reference in emergency situations. These detailed information sheets are also a good periodic refresher source for the perioperative nurse.

SUMMARY

There are many options and considerations in the choice of anesthetic agent and technique to facilitate ambulatory surgery. The goal is to provide the most pleasant and safe experience for the patient. Therefore, to best provide quality postoperative care, it is essential that the nurse understand the postoperative differences to be expected during recovery from the various types of anesthesia.

EXAM QUESTIONS

CHAPTER 3

Questions 18-39

Note: Choose the option that BEST answers each question.

18. A possible side effect of premedication with a benzodiazepine is

    a. nausea.
    b. dizziness.
    c. extrapyramidal stimulation.
    d. seizures.

19. A drug that accelerates gastric emptying is

    a. ondansetron (Zofran).
    b. droperidol (Inapsine).
    c. metoclopramide (Reglan).
    d. glycopyrrolate (Robinul).

20. A state of controlled unconscious analgesia describes

    a. conscious sedation.
    b. general anesthesia.
    c. regional anesthesia.
    d. twilight sedation.

21. The three major phases of general anesthesia are

    a. induction, delirium, and recovery.
    b. delirium, maintenance, and recovery.
    c. induction, maintenance, and recovery.
    d. delirium, depression, and recovery.

22. The only inhalation anesthetic that is a gas at room temperature is

    a. halothane (Fluothane).
    b. succinylcholine.
    c. desflurane (Suprane).
    d. nitrous oxide.

23. An agent that increases the sensitivity of the heart to the dysrhythmic effects of epinephrine is

    a. halothane.
    b. succinylcholine.
    c. desflurane.
    d. nitrous oxide.

24. Because of the strong alkalinity of thiopental (Pentothal) and methohexital (Brevital), precautions should be taken to prevent

    a. regurgitation.
    b. aspiration.
    c. extravasation.
    d. contamination.

25. Rapid recovery characterized by clearheadedness is a characteristic of

    a. etomidate (Amidate).
    b. methohexital.
    c. propofol (Diprivan).
    d. thiopental.

26. The agent with the highest incidence of postoperative nausea and vomiting is

pg39

a. etomidate.
b. methohexital.
c. propofol.
d. thiopental.

27. An agent that may be given intramuscularly to induce anesthesia is

a. etomidate.
b. propofol.
c. desflurane.
d. ketamine.

pg37 & 40

28. Drugs used to paralyze skeletal muscles are

a. tranquilizers.
b. benzodiazepines.
c. local anesthetics.
d. neuromuscular blocking agents.

pg 40-41

29. An atypically low level of plasma cholinesterase will

a. trigger malignant hyperthermia.
b. prolong the effect of succinylcholine.
c. trigger porphyria.
d. shorten the effect of succinylcholine.

pg 41

30. Inducing loss of sensation in a specific area of the body results in what type of anesthesia?

a. Inhalation
b. Regional
c. Intravenous
d. Neuromuscular

pg42

31. After the anesthetic has been injected into the cerebrospinal fluid (CSF), which parameter is extremely important in controlling the level of spinal anesthesia that develops?

pg44

a. Position of the patient
b. IV infusion rate
c. Supplemental oxygen
d. Blood pressure level

32. Leakage of CSF from the puncture in the dura mater made by the spinal needle may result in

a. chemical neuropathy.
b. cerebrovascular accident.
c. spinal cord herniation.
d. postdural puncture headache.

pg45

33. Spread of local anesthetic to the femoral nerve after an ilioinguinal nerve block may delay discharge due to

a. nausea and vomiting.
b. hypotension.
c. systemic toxicity.
d. difficulty in walking.

pg47

34. A patient who has received a local anesthetic begins to shake uncontrollably. The cause is most likely

pg49

a. delayed anxiety.
b. allergic reaction.
c. central nervous system (CNS) toxicity.
d. repressed anger.

35. A large total dose of local anesthetic is less likely to cause CNS toxicity if the patient has been premedicated with a

pg50

a. phenothiazine.
b. narcotic.
c. benzodiazepine.
d. butyrophenone.

36. The medication of choice for the treatment of CNS toxicity due to a local anesthetic is IV

    a. thiopental.
    b. diazepam (Valium).
    c. phenytoin (Dilantin).
    d. propofol.

37. Addition of a vasoconstrictor to the local anesthetic will

    a. reduce the duration of effect.
    b. prolong the duration of effect.
    c. increase toxicity.
    d. increase tissue absorption.

38. After the injection of a local anesthetic with epinephrine, the patient complains of headache and palpitations. The nurse should suspect

    a. allergic reaction.
    b. CNS toxicity.
    c. reaction to epinephrine.
    d. cerebrovascular accident.

39. Documentation of monitoring of the patient who has received a local anesthetic drug should

    a. be done for 15 minutes after the administration.
    b. be done if a systemic reaction if suspected.
    c. provide evidence of continuous assessment.
    d. not include nursing interventions.

CHAPTER 4

PROCEDURAL SEDATION

CHAPTER OBJECTIVE

Upon completion of this chapter, the reader will will be able to discuss the role and responsibilities of the perioperative nurse in the care of patients receiving procedural sedation.

LEARNING OBJECTIVES

After studying this chapter, the reader will be able to

1. define the concept of procedural sedation.
2. identify the pharmacologic agents used to produce moderate sedation.
3. recognize the necessity of vigilant patient monitoring during sedation.
4. describe strategies for patent airway maintenance.

INTRODUCTION

Procedural sedation utilizes a pharmacologically induced state of sedation, with or without analgesia (sedation/analgesia), that facilitates patient comfort and acceptance during appropriate surgical procedures. Note legal scope-of-practice issues concerning procedural sedation are defined by individual state statutes and administered by state boards of nursing. Many state boards of nursing have formal policy statements that define the responsibilities of the registered nurse relative to sedation procedures. The information provided in this chapter relates to nurse and anesthesiologist administered sedation. National and state guidelines as well as facility policies and professional standards should be considered for the appropriateness of the provider in individual situations.

PROCEDURAL SEDATION

Moderate, or procedural, sedation is a term used to describe a state of minimally depressed consciousness wherein the patient independently maintains airway control and responds appropriately to physical stimulation and verbal commands. It is a pharmacologically induced depression of consciousness, with or without analgesia that facilitates patient comfort and acceptance during appropriate surgical procedures.

Most patients are concerned about pain and awareness during surgery under local anesthesia, yet they would prefer not to undergo general anesthesia. With the judicious use of sedation and analgesia, the patient objectives of relief of anxiety, prevention of pain, and enhanced cooperation can be achieved with minimal risk.

Induced sedation is a continuum identifiable by four levels: minimal (anxiolysis), moderate (procedural), deep, and then general anesthesia. (See Table 4-1.) The Joint Commission includes these four

TABLE 4-1: CONTINUUM OF DEPTH OF SEDATION LEVELS OF SEDATION/ANALGESIA

	Minimal Sedation (Anxiolysis)	*Moderate Sedation / Analgesia ("Conscious Sedation")*	*Deep Sedation / Analgesia*	*General Anesthesia*
Responsiveness	Normal response to verbal stimulation	Purposeful response to verbal or tactile stimulation	Purposeful response following repeated or painful stimulation	Unarousable even with painful stimulus
Airway	Unaffected	No intervention required	Intervention may be required	Intervention often required
Spontaneous Ventilation	Unaffected	Adequate	May be inadequate	Frequently inadequate
Cardiovascular Function	Unaffected	Usually maintained	Usually maintained	May be impaired

Note. From "Practice Guidelines for Sedation and Analgesia by Non-Anesthesiologists, An Updated Report by the American Society of Anesthesiologists Task Force on Sedation and Analgesia by Non-Anesthesiologists," 2002, *Anesthesiology, 96*: 1004-17. Retrieved November 26, 2008, from http://www.asahq.org/publicationsAndServices/sedation1017.pdf. Reprinted with permission.

levels in their standards. During minimal sedation the patient responds normally. During moderate or procedural sedation/analgesia the patient responds purposefully to verbal or tactile stimulation and the airway and cardiovascular system are maintained. In deep sedation/analgesia the patient responds purposefully only following repeated or painful stimulation and may lose protective reflexes and may not be able to maintain the airway. At the level of general anesthesia, consciousness and the ability to move are lost, the patient is unable to respond even to painful stimulation, and may not be able to maintain the airway (American Association of Nurse Anesthetists [AANA], 2003; American Society of Anesthesiologists [ASA], 2002).

The medications, doses, and techniques used for procedural sedation are not intended to produce unconsciousness; the goal is to use as little medication as possible to make the patient as comfortable as possible and to do so as safely as possible. Adequate sedation may be identified by a calm demeanor, slurred speech, slowed heart rate, or reduced blood pressure. Incremental drug administration until the patient's eyes close spontaneously usually signifies adequate anxiolytic effect and amnesia (Conahan & Young, 1997). A sedated patient whose only response is reflex withdrawal from painful stimuli is sedated beyond the level of procedural sedation (AANA, 2003; ASA, 2002).

Deep sedation may be accompanied by a partial or complete loss of protective reflexes, the inability to manage oropharyngeal secretions, or an inability to continuously maintain a patent airway, leading to possible aspiration and hypoxia. Other complications of deep sedation include hypotension, hypoventilation, respiratory depression, and apnea.

Used in conjunction with local or regional anesthesia, procedural sedation may obviate the need for general anesthesia and its associated physiologic effects for appropriate surgical procedures. Patients with significant anxiety or previous unpleasant general anesthetic experiences are candidates for this technique for ambulatory surgery. In children and uncooperative adults, the use of procedural sedation may facilitate diagnostic procedures that require the patient not to move.

Sedation should not be extended beyond safe limits to facilitate a failed regional anesthetic. When the basic regional technique does not provide complete anesthesia, the procedure should be postponed or the patient should be given a general anesthetic, if appropriate (Chung & Lam, 1997). To obtain optimal patient safety and comfort, careful titration of sedative and analgesic drugs; vigilant monitoring of the cardiovascular, respiratory, and neurologic systems; and effective communication with both the patient and surgeon are necessary (Sweitzer, 1998). The facility should have written guidelines for the administration of procedural sedation that include dosage and monitoring parameters plus reversal and resuscitation protocols (O'Donnell, Bragg, & Sell, 2003).

PATIENT SELECTION

Appropriate patient selection is essential to ensure a safe and effective procedure (Shankar & Deshpande, 2005). Using the ASA classification of physical status, class P1 and P2 and selected class P3 and P4 patients are appropriate candidates for sedation (Sweitzer, 1998). However, patients with severe cardiac, pulmonary, hepatic, renal, or central nervous system (CNS) disease; morbid obesity; or sleep apnea are at increased risk for developing complications related to sedation/analgesia unless special precautions are taken. Pregnancy, drug or alcohol abuse, extremes of age and uncooperative patients also require special precautions.

Risks may be reduced by consultation with appropriate specialists before the procedure. In cases where sedation to the point of unresponsiveness or general anesthesia may become necessary, monitoring by an anesthesia provider is appropriate (ASA, 2006). Consequently, final patient selection is considerably dependent on thorough patient assessment.

PATIENT ASSESSMENT

All of the criteria relevant to preoperative assessment for general anesthesia are relevant to procedural sedation. The importance of family history and the patient's own prior experience with sedation, analgesia, and anesthesia should not be overlooked. A factual history of drug and alcohol usage is especially important for this technique.

The Association of periOperative Registered Nurses (AORN) recommends that candidates for moderate sedation be assessed physiologically and psychologically prior to the procedures to provide baseline data and identify risk factors. Age, weight, physical status, and psychologic predisposition are important influences on sensitivity to sedative and analgesic medications. All assessment results should be documented.

In females of childbearing age the possibility of pregnancy must be considered. If possible, pregnancy should be confirmed or ruled out. At least the date of the last menstrual period should be documented. Clinicians at each facility should determine and set clear guidelines or policy on pre-sedation pregnancy testing.

Because of the inherent danger of deep sedation, which causes loss of adequate airway control, obstruction may occur during spontaneous respiration when airway abnormalities are present. Any anomaly or physical condition that would adversely affect instituting and maintaining a patent airway and positive pressure ventilation should be closely examined, documented, and brought to the attention of the surgeon prior to administering any medication. Table 4-2 describes factors that may be associated with difficulty in airway management.

Physical conditions that could affect the airway would include any condition that impedes neck extension or forward and upward movement of the jaw; all potential problems should be noted and appraised. A short neck, receding chin, or small mouth may present problems. Limited neck extension due to arthritis, disease or trauma of the cervical spine, or scarring of the skin over the throat are examples that may cause major problems should manual airway control or tracheal intubation become necessary.

Management of the obese patient's airway during procedural sedation may be problematic because of increased body mass and redundant

TABLE 4-2: EXAMPLE OF AIRWAY ASSESSMENT PROCEDURES FOR SEDATION AND ANALGESIA
Positive-pressure ventilation, with or without endotracheal intubation, may be necessary if respiratory compromise develops during sedation/analgesia. This intervention may be more difficult in patients with atypical airway anatomy. Also, some airway abnormalities may increase the likelihood of airway obstruction during spontaneous ventilation. Some factors that may be associated with difficulty in airway management are:
History
Previous problems with anesthesia or sedation
Stridor, snoring, or sleep apnea
Advanced rheumatoid arthritis
Chromosomal abnormality (e.g., trisomy 21)
Physical Examination
Habitus
Significant obesity (especially involving the neck and facial structures)
Head and Neck
Short neck, limited neck extension, decreased hyoid-mental distance (less than 3 cm in an adult), neck mass, cervical spine disease or trauma, tracheal deviation, dysmorphic facial features (e.g., Pierre-Robin syndrome)
Mouth
Small opening (less than 3 cm in an adult), edentulous mouth, protruding incisors, loose or capped teeth, presence of dental appliances, high arched palate, macroglossia, tonsillar hypertrophy, nonvisible uvula
Jaw
Micrognathia, retrognathia, trismus, significant malocclusion
Note. From "Practice Guidelines for Sedation and Analgesia by Non-Anesthesiologists, An Updated Report by the American Society of Anesthesiologists Task Force on Sedation and Analgesia by Non-Anesthesiologists," 2002, *Anesthesiology, 96*: 1004-17. Retrieved November 26, 2008, from http://www.asahq.org/publicationsAndServices/sedation1017.pdf. Reprinted with permission.

oropharyngeal tissue. For these patients, the level of sedation must be carefully titrated. Because obese patients are prone to pulmonary aspiration secondary to increased gastric volume and gastric reflux, the preoperative administration of histamine-2 blockers, such as ranitidine (Zantac) or cimetidine (Tagamet), and gastric stimulants, such as metoclopramide (Reglan, Octamide, Maxolon), may be of benefit (Kost, 2004).

Dentition should be examined and documented in detail, both for the patient's safety and medicolegal reasons. Loose teeth, chipped teeth, missing teeth, and cosmetic dental appliances are important findings to be documented on the patient's record preoperatively. Not only are these factors important if an oropharyngeal airway or endotracheal intubation becomes necessary, but very loose teeth may become dislodged and possibly aspirated from other manipulations. Dentures and partial dentures should be removed, but in elderly patients with flaccid facial tissue, a better airway may be maintained if the dentures are in place. Whether to remove dentures must be decided on an individual basis, discussed with the patient, and documented.

The preprocedure assessment should include a minimum of a physical examination and a focused history that lists current medications including alternative or complimentary herbal medications and over-the-counter products. The sedation provider should be familiar with the interactions between these drugs, between these drugs and the sedative/analgesia medications to be used, and the possible effect with the procedural sedation, such as increased bleeding tendency.

Allergies or problems related to previous procedures or medications should be defined. A history of snoring, sleep apnea, smoking, or alcohol or drug abuse is important not only for choosing the pharmacologic agents to be used, but to assist in determining the cause of any untoward event that may occur during the procedure or recovery.

PREOPERATIVE PREPARATION

Ideally, a patient-specific procedural sedation plan will have been developed for each patient and communicated among the procedure team (Shankar & Deshpande, 2005). Timely appropriate laboratory tests should be on the chart, and any medications ordered for preoperative administration, such as antibiotics, should have been documented (O'Donnell, Bragg, & Sell, 2003). Last intake of fluids and food should be verified and documented.

One of the most beneficial preoperative procedures is establishing rapport with the patient. This relationship can significantly reduce the patient's anxiety and facilitate communication between the patient and person monitoring the sedation during the procedure.

The patient's personal concerns should be explored and discussed, taking into consideration cultural and societal influences. Care should be taken to clearly answer patient questions, but detailed explanations do not seem to reduce anxiety more than brief explanations (Sweitzer, 1998). Technical discussions may actually increase anxiety.

Patients, or their legal guardians in the case of minors or legally incompetent adults, should be informed about and agree to the administration of sedatives and analgesic medications before any medication is given. Risks, alternatives, and benefits should be explained before consent is obtained. A separate procedural sedation consent is advisable, but a defined area on the operative consent form that specifically addresses the risks, alternatives, and benefits associated with intravenous (IV) sedation is also acceptable (Kost, 2004). Informed consent should be documented on the patient's chart according to the facility's policy (Shankar & Deshpande, 2005).

Preprocedure fasting should be ordered for the patient receiving procedural sedation. Circumstances such as an inadequate regional block, a surgical procedure that outlasts the duration of the block, or drug idiosyncrasy may necessitate a transition to the use of general anesthesia. Although there is considerable difference of opinion on the duration for which the patient should not have ingested food or liquids (i.e., nothing by mouth [NPO]), a generalization for the healthy adult is to allow a light meal of tea and toast up to 6 hours before surgery. Preferably the toast should be lightly buttered or unbuttered. Other options include crackers, sugar cookies, and gelatin. Fruit juice may be allowed if it is without pulp. Solid foods should be withheld for longer durations. Gastric emptying is slowest with fats, intermediate with carbohydrates, and fastest with protein-rich food (Pandit, 2000). Table 4-3 provides a protocol on fasting recommended by the ASA.

Children are allowed clear liquids until 2 hours before the procedure. Due to high fat content, breast milk or formula is generally permitted only until 4 hours prior to the procedure. It is important to remember that fear, obesity, pain, opioids, pregnancy, and conditions associated with abnormal autonomic function, such as diabetes, are some of the conditions that may decrease gastric emptying (Riley, 2003).

Prior to the administration of any medication or surgical preparation, it should be established that the patient is not wearing contact lenses. Those who wear contact lenses routinely neglect to mention them. But should the use of an oxygen mask become necessary, severe corneal abrasions may occur if contact lenses are left in the eyes.

TABLE 4-3: SUMMARY OF AMERICAN SOCIETY OF ANESTHESIOLOGISTS PREPROCEDURE FASTING GUIDELINES

Ingested Material	Minimum Fasting Period†
Clear liquids‡	2 hours
Breast milk	4 hours
Infant formula	6 hours
Nonhuman milk§	6 hours
Light meal*	6 hours

These recommendations apply to healthy patients who are undergoing elective procedures. They are not intended for women in labor. Following the Guidelines does not guarantee a complete gastric emptying has occurred.

† The fasting periods apply to all ages.

‡ Examples of clear liquids include water, fruit juices without pulp, carbonated beverages, clear tea, and black coffee.

§ Since nonhuman milk is similar to solids in gastric emptying time, the amount ingested must be considered when determining an appropriate fasting period.

* A light meal typically consists of toast and clear liquids. Meals that include fried or fatty foods or meat may prolong gastric emptying time. Both the amount and type of foods ingested must be considered when determining an appropriate fasting period.

Note. From "Practice Guidelines for Sedation and Analgesia by Non-Anesthesiologists, An Updated Report by the American Society of Anesthesiologists Task Force on Sedation and Analgesia by Non-Anesthesiologists," 2002, *Anesthesiology, 96*: 1004-17. Retrieved November 26, 2008, from http://www.asahq.org/publicationsAndServices/sedation1017.pdf. Reprinted with permission.

PREMEDICATION

The purpose of premedication is to reduce apprehension and anxiety. Benzodiazepines are well suited to this purpose and may be taken orally prior to arrival at the facility, if appropriate. However, taking benzodiazepines in advance may compromise the patient's safety because of the possibility of dizziness or difficulty walking. Still, it is important that the medication be taken in sufficient time to allow maximum effect to be attained well before the start of the procedure; such timing prevents unanticipated additive effects during operative administration of sedation.

If indicated, antiemetics, such as ondansetron and transdermal scopolamine may be taken before arrival at the facility because they do not cause sedation (Dershwitz, 1998). Children older than 3 years are candidates for liquid oral benzodiazepine premedication. The medicine may be distasteful, but it may be given with a minimal amount of sweet liquid. Suitable premedication relieves anxiety and produces mild sedation, resulting in a cooperative patient. Premedication was discussed more fully in Chapter 3.

INTRAOPERATIVE MEDICATIONS

Desirable pharmacologic characteristics for producing procedural sedation include rapid onset of action, short duration of action, lack of cumulative effects, minimal side effects, and rapid metabolization. Because sedation and analgesia may be required to achieve a relaxed, pain-free state of detachment, a combination of medications is often necessary.

Sedatives are pharmacologic agents that reduce anxiety (anxiolytics) and may cause some degree of amnesia and alteration of time perception. Analgesics reduce or ameliorate pain perception. Combining different types of medications may require lower doses of each drug because of possible synergistic effect, although the risk of respiratory depression, hypotension, and prolonged sedation is increased. Additionally, should reversal be necessary, it may be difficult to establish which medication caused the unwanted effect (O'Donnell, Bragg, & Sell, 2003)

Ameliorate - make something bad or unsatisfactory better.

Benzodiazepines

Benzodiazepines have become the class of drugs most widely used for procedural sedation. They produce dose-related sedation, anxiolytic effects, and amnesia. Benzodiazepines have no analgesic properties. They may be used in conjunction with analgesic medications, but the use of opioids prolongs recovery times. Patient response to this pharmacologic category is widely variable, and drug dosage must be carefully titrated, as well as reduced for elderly patients. When benzodiazepines are used to produce profound sedation, amnesia may occur for events during the early postoperative recovery period.

Diazepam (Valium)

Diazepam has been widely used for procedural sedation and is particularly useful with regional anesthesia because it exerts the strongest anticonvulsant effect of all the benzodiazepines by increasing the seizure threshold for local anesthetics. When administered IV, sedation usually occurs within 2 to 3 minutes; subsequent doses should be given no less than 3 minutes apart.

Diazepam should not be considered a drug of short duration. Following a period of apparent recovery, drowsiness and an increase in plasma concentration have been reported at 6 to 8 hours, probably due to intrahepatic recirculation (Morgan, Mikahil, & Murray, 2006). By the same mechanism, an increase in serum concentration resulting in an increase in drowsiness may occur when fatty foods are consumed 3 to 7 hours after administration of diazepam. Fatty foods should be restricted during the recovery period to avoid resedation, especially when a large total dosage has been given. Age decreases the clearance of diazepam whereas smoking increases its clearance (Reves, Glass, Lubarsky, & McEvoy, 2005).

Ambulatory patients should also be cautioned that they may feel tired for a day or more after receiving IV diazepam. With large doses, impairment of coordination and reactive skills may persist for 10 hours. Pain during IV injection and possible postprocedure phlebitis caused by the propylene glycol required in parentral preparations, are major drawbacks. Using larger veins and reducing the rate of injection may help to alleviate pain and sequelae. Restricting the use of diazepam to oral premedication may be an option.

Cimetidine reduces the metabolism of diazepam, while 1000 units of heparin may increase diazepam concentration as much as 200% (Morgan, Mikhail, & Murray, 2006).

Midazolam (Versed)

Because midazolam is prepared in an aqueous solution, it causes minimal venous irritation. It has a faster onset of action (1 to 2 minutes) and provides more effective amnesia than diazepam. It is three to six times as potent as diazepam (Reves et al., 2005). Because midazolam does not undergo intrahepatic recirculation, drowsiness does not usually recur after the patient recovers; however, large doses may cause prolonged drowsiness. Unlike diazepam and lorazepam, midazolam has not been approved for oral administration in the United States.

Midazolam's rapid onset and redistribution have made it a popular choice for procedures involving procedural sedation, but it should be given in small increments, with sufficient time allowed for its effect to develop, until signs such as slurred speech and drooping eyelids occur. Midazolam's high potency requires careful titration to avoid overdosage and apnea (Morgan, Mikhail, & Murray, 2006). Depending on the patient's general condition, drug history, and alcohol use, response is variable. Elderly patients require lower doses (Reves et al., 2005).

Midazolam is pharmacologically suitable for continuous infusion administration, but careful titration is necessary. Administration must be terminated soon enough to avoid excessive sedation and prolonged recovery. Early in its clinical usage, midazolam was associated with a significant number of incidences of respiratory depression, apnea, cardiac arrests, and deaths. Most of these involved elderly patients undergoing endoscopic procedures without dedicated monitoring (Sweitzer, 1998). However, for all patients, respiratory depression is the most significant adverse event associated with midazolam (Reves et al., 2005)

Renal disease or failure may lead to prolonged sedation with midazolam due to the accumulation of a conjugated metabolite. Benzodiazepines as a group generally support cardiovascular hemodynamics, although midazolam tends to lower blood pressure more than diazepam (Morgan, Mikhail, & Murray, 2006).

Sensations of pressure, movement, or visceral traction sometimes experienced by patients under various types of regional block may be reduced with concomitant analgesic therapy. Similarly, if the block proves inadequate or the duration of surgery outlasts the effectiveness of the regional block, narcotics may be required to keep the patient comfortable, but combining a narcotic with a benzodiazepine lowers blood pressure and increases respiratory depression more than each drug would do individually (Reves et al., 2005).

Opioids

Fentanyl (Sublimaze)

Fentanyl, a potent narcotic congener of meperidine, is widely used in ambulatory settings. After IV administration, response usually begins within 2 minutes and lasts 45 to 60 minutes. With a redistribution half-life of 13.4 minutes, 98.6% of the injected dose is cleared from the plasma in 60 minutes. This rapid clearance makes it useful for outpatient sedation.

Although fentanyl is considered appropriate for ambulatory surgery, it can produce marked respiratory depression. Care should be taken to avoid a dosage sufficient to produce a sleeplike state in which there is a lack of spontaneous verbalization. This sleeplike state has been identified as one of the recurring problems found in unexpected cardiac arrests during spinal anesthesia. Cyanosis frequently heralded the onset of cardiac arrest in patients exhibiting this degree of sedation, which suggests that undetected respiratory insufficiency may have played an important role. Diazepam and droperidol have also been implicated in similar situations.

Fentanyl is often given in combination with a benzodiazepine, which significantly increases respiratory depression compared to either drug used alone. Because fentanyl has some sedative effect in addition to its narcotic effect, combination with a benzodiazepine produces more profound sedation and improved patient cooperation than does a benzodiazepine alone (Sweitzer, 1998).

Appropriate monitoring is essential for the patient's safety. If fentanyl is injected too rapidly, chest rigidity may occur (Shankar & Deshpande, 2005). Fentanyl is not recommended for patients who have taken monoamine oxidase inhibitors within 14 days (Pasero, 2006).

Alfentanil (Alfenta)

The opioids alfentanil, sufentanil, and remifentanil are typically administered by an anesthesia provider in a monitored anesthesia care situation. Their potency and potentially lethal side effects if improperly administered or monitored make these drugs dangerous in less skilled hands.

Alfentanil is a short-acting fentanyl analog with one quarter the potency and one third the duration of fentanyl. Nevertheless, large doses may result in prolonged sedation and respiratory depression. Compared with fentanyl, alfentanil produces more hypotension and more muscular rigidity if administered too rapidly, although fentanyl, sufentanil, and alfentanil may cause rigidity severe enough to prevent sufficient ventilation (Morgan, Mikhail, & Murray, 2006).

The pharmacokinetics of alfentanil suggests that it may be best administered by continuous infusion; the ability to closely titrate dosage is a major advantage of this technique. By using a continuous infusion, the total amount of narcotic administered may be decreased significantly. Although discharge may be delayed because of postoperative nausea and vomiting with alfentanil or fentanyl use, less nausea and vomiting is associated with alfentanil (Tesniere & Servin, 2003).

Sufentanil (Sufenta)

Sufentanil is shorter acting than alfentanil and extremely potent. It is eight to ten times as potent as fentanyl but otherwise pharmacokinetically very similar (Jablonka & Davis, 2005). When administered by continuous IV infusion for procedures of intermediate duration, recovery should be almost 50% more rapid. However, compared to maintenance by intermittent boluses, IV infusion may result in episodes of hypoxemia (Tesniere & Servin, 2003).

Remifentanil (Ultiva)

Remifentanil is an ultra short-acting opioid. Because it is so rapidly metabolized, it is typically administered by using a loading dose, then continuous IV infusion. Regardless of total dosage or duration of administration, recovery is rapid and may be expected within 5 to 10 minutes after the drug is discontinued. If significant postoperative pain is expected, remifentanil may not be an appropriate opioid choice. However, an alternative is the multimodal administration of nonopiod analgesics well before remifentanil is discontinued. Because of its kinetic predictability and maintenance of cardiovascular stability, remifentanil has become a useful choice for pediatric analgesia and anesthesia (Jablonka & Davis, 2005)

Morphine Sulfate and Meperidine (Demerol)

These classic opiate and opioid examples are poor choices for procedural sedation unless extended duration of effect is desirable. In the absence of pain, long-acting morphine may cause significant dysphoria. In small doses, meperidine produces pleasant euphoria and has a duration between that of morphine and fentanyl, but it may cause abnormal coordination and reaction for up to 12 hours. Morphine sulfate and meperidine cause more nausea, vomiting, dizziness, and a longer duration of respiratory depression than shorter acting opioids (Sweitzer, 1998).

Agonist-Antagonist Opioids

In an attempt to achieve analgesia with fewer side effects, agonist-antagonists such as butorphanol (Stadol) and nalbuphine (Nubain) were developed. Administered independently, this class of drugs produces opioid effects but antagonizes the effects of full agonists if given with them. These agents may trigger withdrawal symptoms in patients with a history of drug abuse.

Butorphanol has an analgesic potency five times that of morphine, whereas nalbuphine is considered equipotent to morphine. Both drugs have sedative effects as well. Their onsets of action occur within 2 minutes after IV administration, but their durations, like that of morphine, are long. Some studies document the recovery time as 1 to 2 hours for butorphanol and consider the postoperative analgesia an asset. Realistically, their recovery time should be 3 to 4 hours, and their use should be restricted to procedures where considerable postoperative pain is anticipated.

Sedative-Hypnotic Agents

These drugs, also referred to as rapid-acting IV induction agents, may be more applicable to monitored anesthesia care (MAC). Although the term MAC is sometimes used interchangeably with procedural sedation, as the name implies, an anesthesia provider monitors the patient, ready to institute general anesthesia if necessary.

The line between sedation and unconsciousness is narrow and occurs quickly with sedative-hypnotic agents. Consequently, the maker of propofol, AstraZeneca Pharmaceuticals (2005), states in the warnings section of the package insert that propofol should be "administered only by persons trained in the administration of general anesthesia and not involved in the conduct of the surgical or diagnostic procedure. Patients should be continuously monitored and facilities for maintenance of a patent airway, artificial ventilation, and oxygen enrichment and circulatory resuscitation must be immediately available".

The Joint Commission stipulates that individuals who administer procedural or deep sedation must be competent to perform the rescues listed in their sedation and anesthesia standards; the availability of a code team is no substitute (Semo, 2005). In 2004, the ASA and the AANA issued a joint statement in accordance with the statements in the package insert. Similarly, the American Association for the Accreditation of Ambulatory Surgical Facilities (AAAASF) states that propofol should only be administered by an anesthesiologist or nurse anesthetist.

Propofol (Diprivan)

Propofol is classified as a sedative-hypnotic without analgesic effect or amnesic properties when given in doses that do not produce unconsciousness. It has gained popularity because it results in rapid recovery with few side effects. Patients quickly appear alert and clearheaded; some experience a significant sense of well-being. Propofol is also believed to have some antiemetic effects and the incidence of postoperative nausea and vomiting is low.

Propofol may be given as an initial bolus or titrated to effect, but it causes pain on injection. This pain may be decreased by using a larger vein, injecting lidocaine before propofol, or adding lidocaine to the propofol solution. Propofol's rapid elimination and lack of cumulative effect make it especially suitable for continuous infusion. Usually, recovery occurs within 3 to 10 minutes regardless of the duration or total dosage. To minimize undesirable cardiorespiratory depression in elderly or debilitated patients, rapid single or repeated bolus administration is not advised. For elderly patients, the initial dose of propofol should be reduced by 40% for procedural sedation (Tesniere & Servin, 2005).

Propofol causes less postoperative sedation, drowsiness, and confusion than midazolam, yet when given alone, it may cause dysphoria. When midazolam is given preoperatively or at the start of the procedure with propofol, it does not delay rapid recovery nor cause additional side effects. This combined usage takes advantage of the rapid recovery associated with propofol as well as midazolam's ability to provide relief from anxiety and amnesia during the procedure (Sweitzer, 1998).

It should be noted that propofol solution provides an excellent medium for bacterial growth. For procedural sedation or general anesthesia, a single syringe or vial of propofol should be discarded within 6 hours of opening (Meyer, 2007; Morgan, Mikhail, & Murray, 2006). The U.S. Food and Drug Administration (FDA) also stipulates that for sedation on the intensive care unit there should be an individual vial used for each patient, which must be discarded after 12 hours.

Methohexital (Brevital)

Methohexital is an ultra short-acting barbiturate also of the group known as IV anesthetics. Widely used as an IV induction agent to produce unconsciousness quickly, it may also be administered by continuous infusion, which results in a reasonably short recovery period. Because it is strongly alkaline, methohexital should be given cautiously to avoid extravasations. Methohexital is closely related to thiopental (Pentothal), but despite its shorter recovery profile, methohexital is more potent. Methohexital is also associated with hiccupping and involuntary movements.

Ketamine (Ketalar)

Ketamine is unique in that it can be administered by the intramuscular (IM) or IV route, which makes it useful in circumstances where IM administration prior to the procedure may be an advantage. However, ketamine produces a dissociative state with undesirable emergence side effects, especially in adults, such as disorientation, hypersensitivity, vivid dreams, and tachycardia. When combined with a benzodiazepine, these psychomimetic reactions and these cardiostimulatory effects may be attenuated. Ketamine also is associated with excessive salivation and airway secretions, producing a risk of aspiration (Shankar & Deshpande, 2005).

Attenuated - to reduce the severity.

Droperidol (Inapsine)

Droperidol, a butyrophenone derivative, has been used for many years as a supplement to surgical and diagnostic procedures. It provides sedation and a sense of detachment with minimal amnesia. When combined with a narcotic, neuroleptanalgesia (i.e., dissociative analgesia) results. Although it does not cause significant respiratory depression, droperidol in large doses may cause hypotension, extrapyramidal effects, and confusion. Overenthusiastic use of droperidol, alone or in neuroleptanalgesia combinations, has generated many reports of complications (Martinez, Moos, & Dahlen, 2006). Droperidol carries a "black box" warning – the most serious warning for a FDA approved drug – because of its association with fatal cardiac dysrhythmias.

Additionally, although clinical recovery from droperidol occurs after 25 minutes, tiredness or drowsiness persists, and tests of coordination and attention remain significantly abnormal after 10 hours. Droperidol is a potent antiemetic, and small doses may be used prophylactically to reduce the incidence of postoperative vomiting in adults and children. Large doses, alone or in combination with fentanyl, are generally considered inappropriate for ambulatory patients. The sedation far outlasts the effect of the narcotic component.

Antagonists

Naloxone (Narcan)

Naloxone reverses CNS) and respiratory depressant effects of narcotics in a dose-dependent manner by competitively binding at receptor sites in the brain and spinal column. It is usually administered IV in small, repeated doses until the desired effect is achieved. CNS effects may be seen in 1 to 2 minutes. Naloxone is an emergency drug and should be immediately available wherever opioids are administered.

However, the reversal procedure should be done cautiously because abrupt reversal may result in sudden pain perception, causing hypertension and tachycardia. Caution should also be used in patients with cardiac disease or suspected or known narcotic dependence.

Flumazenil (Romazicon)

Flumazenil works by displacing benzodiazepines at their receptor sites. Therefore, it does not reverse the effects of drugs which bind elsewhere, such as barbiturates, antidepressants, alcohol, or general anesthesia. Given IV, flumazenil's onset of action occurs in 1 to 2 minutes, with peak effect in 6 to 10 minutes.

The half-life of flumazenil is 41 to 79 minutes. Except for midazolam, most benzodiazepines have a longer half-life than flumazenil, so patients should be monitored for resedation for up to 2 hours. Flumazenil-induced seizures have been reported in patients treated with benzodiazepines to control seizures and in patients with chronic physical dependence on these drugs. Pain at the injection site sometimes occurs, and flumazenil has been associated with thrombophlebitis.

Flumazenil is effective in reversing drug-induced sedation and respiratory depression when only benzodiazepines have been administered. In patients who have received both opioids and benzodiazepines, flumazenil is known to reverse benzodiazepine-induced sedation; however, its effectiveness in reversing respiratory depression under these circumstances is unclear.

TECHNIQUES OF ADMINISTRATION

Usually, sedation is administered IV; therefore, IV access should be maintained throughout the procedure and until there is no longer a risk of respiratory depression occurring after the stimulation of the procedure has ended. Existing IV access is an important safety feature should an emergency situation develop.

In cases where the medications for sedation/analgesia were administered nonintravenously, or where the IV line has become blocked or infiltration has occurred, the decision to establish or reestablish IV access should be made on a case-by-case basis, with an individual skilled in IV insertion immediately available (Association of Operating Room Nurses [AORN], 2006; ASA, 2002).

Incremental Single-Dose Injection

Incremental single-dose injection, also referred to as titration to effect, involves the administration of small, incremental IV doses of sedative/analgesic medications until the optimal level of effect is achieved. Subsequent doses are given as needed during the procedure to maintain this level. Incremental titration improves the margin of safety for sedation, but care must be taken to allow sufficient time for each dose to become fully effective before additional increments are given.

When a sedative and an analgesic drug are used, studies suggest that the safest method is to administer each component separately. Thus the sedative would be titrated slowly until the desired level of anxiety reduction or decreased awareness is achieved, and the analgesia would be incrementally administered until relief of discomfort is achieved.

Fixed combinations of sedative and analgesic given simultaneously may increase the possibility of adverse events, such as respiratory and cardiac depression. Total dosage of medication is often greater because two drugs must be administered when only one effect, either sedation or analgesia, may be needed. Not only is this less cost-effective, but an increased amount of medication must be metabolized, which may result in prolonged recovery.

To establish an analgesic base, opioids are sometimes administered before benzodiazepines. If given IM rather than IV, the narcotic should be given at least 45 to 60 minutes prior to operation. Disadvantages associated with IM narcotic injection include inadvertent injection subcutaneously, which further delays onset of effect; poor absorption; and the necessity of qualified personnel to monitor the patient after the narcotic has been administered (Kost, 2004).

Bolus Injection

With this technique, the total estimated dose, based on patient size, weight, and age, is given in a single injection. The intent is to rapidly achieve a therapeutic plasma concentration just before the start of the procedure. Bolus injection is frequently used for gastroenterologic procedures.

Risks associated with this technique may considerably outweigh the perceived benefits of rapidly producing the desired plasma level needed for effect. This high-risk situation is especially true in elderly patients where reduced total dose, or a percentage of estimated dose, may be advisable to avoid cardiac or respiratory depression or collapse.

Rapid injection of large doses may also cause unconsciousness and muscle rigidity of the chest wall. Small incremental boluses allow the desired plasma level to be produced slowly while potentially using less medication to produce the same pharmacologic effect (Kost, 2004).

Continuous Infusion

Continuous, variable-rate IV infusion facilitates establishing and maintaining a plasma concentration sufficient to produce the necessary level of effect. Initially the level of sedation is achieved by infusing a loading dose of medication over 5 to 15 minutes, which is then maintained by an infusion rate that may be varied to achieve a steady state of patient comfort (Sweitzer, 1998).

Frequently used for the administration of sedative-hypnotic agents (also called IV anesthetics), continuous infusion with proper titration may be associated with less respiratory depression and more rapid recovery. When analgesics are administered using this technique, a more stable level of comfort, fewer side effects, and decreased total dosage may result.

The continuous infusion technique requires a carrier IV solution with the continuous medication infusion piggybacked into the carrier solution. Extreme care must be taken to avoid running the carrier solution at a keep-vein-open or slow rate, which allows a buildup of the infusion medication into the venoset. When the carrier fluid is opened, the patient receives a large bolus of medication which may result in overdose (Kost, 2004). Conversely, it is important not to administer the IV solution used to maintain line patency in a quantity sufficient to stimulate urine production, which would cause overdistention of the bladder and patient discomfort.

MONITORING

Because the use of procedural sedation requires vigilant observation of the patient, ideally the nurse should have no other responsibilities or distractions. AORN guidelines clearly state that the nurse monitoring the patient must be able to immediately recognize and respond to adverse physiologic and psychological changes during the procedures.

The ASA guidelines suggest that the person monitoring the patient may assist with interruptible ancillary tasks of short duration after an adequate and stable level of sedation/analgesia has been achieved so long as adequate monitoring is maintained. These guidelines also contend that having an individual other than the person performing the procedure monitor the patient's status reduces risks and improves patient satisfaction. When sedation is provided by the individual also performing the surgery, as may occur in office-based practices, there is added risk of diverting the operator's attention from the primary focus of performing the procedure (Sweitzer, 1998).

The concept of rescuing the sedated patient who has drifted into a deeper than intended level of sedation has been introduced by The Joint Commission. Therefore, the person administering the sedation or analgesia should be capable of appropriately treating, or rescuing, the patient at any of the four stages of sedation (Shankar & Deshpande, 2005).

Each facility should have written guidelines for the administration of procedural sedation that not only include dosage and monitoring parameters, but reversal and resuscitation protocols as well. These should explicitly define treatment for any patient who loses protective reflexes (Riley, 2003).

Continued emotional support of mentally competent, cooperative adults may reduce the amount of pharmacologic intervention needed. Such support may be provided by reassuring touch and verbal interaction if movement of the face is not contraindicated by the procedure. Verbal response by the patient serves the dual purpose of ensuring that spontaneous breathing is taking place. If verbal response is not appropriate, a gesture of communication established between the patient and the nurse monitor before the start of sedation might be used. Simply asking the patient to take a few deep breaths provides another means of communication that serves dual purposes.

The nurse monitoring the patient should have a thorough understanding of the pharmacology of all medications used to produce sedation/analgesia and the possible complications associated with their use, as well as applicable antagonists and emergency medications. Because most complications associated with procedural sedation involve the cardiorespiratory and neurologic systems, knowledge of the anatomy and physiology of these systems is essential. An understanding of the principles of oxygen delivery, transport, and uptake, plus experience with oxygen delivery devices should be part of the facility's educational/credentialing mechanism of the nurse's competency (AANA, 2003).

The nurse monitor should be able to recognize developing untoward events and be able to immediately intervene appropriately. Skill in airway maintenance and the use of cardiac and respiratory support equipment is required. Advanced cardiac life support (ACLS, PALS) certification is recommended, but requirement for the certification depends on the protocols established by each ambulatory surgery facility. However, someone knowledgeable in life support should be immediately available. For procedural sedation this person or persons should be 1 to 5 minutes away and actually in the procedure room for deep sedation (Shankar & Deshpande, 2005). Noticing and responding to subtle respiratory changes, such as rate, effort, or quality, in patients with chronic obstructive pulmonary disease may prevent the need for rescue treatment (Riley, 2003)

Studies have shown that the use of supplemental oxygen, as opposed to breathing room air, produces decreased incidence and severity of hypoxemia during sedation/analgesia. Although it would seem prudent to administer supplemental oxygen, the decision may be made on a case-by-case basis. It should be noted that by delaying the onset of hypoxemia, supplemental oxygen will delay the detection of apnea by pulse oximetry (Joshi, 2006; Shankar & Deshpande, 2005). This delay emphasizes the need for constant observation of the patient by a well-trained individual rather than relying on monitoring equipment, no matter how sophisticated, during sedation.

With or without supplementation, an oxygen supply and bag-valve mask postive-pressure ventilation system, as well as a source of suction, should be present and, ideally, dedicated to the patient being monitored. The patient should not be given any IV medication if this equipment is not immediately available. In most operating rooms these would be standard pieces of equipment; however, they may not be standard for preoperative holding areas or endoscopy rooms. Table 4-4 lists emergency equipment that should be available. It is important that sizes of equipment appropriate to the patient's physical size be included. The ASA recommends that a defibrillator also be immediately available for patients with significant cardiac disease.

Baseline vital signs should be established and documented prior to the start of sedation, then checked and recorded every 5 minutes during the procedure and at regular intervals until recovery takes place. Vital signs to monitor include blood pressure; pulse rate, rhythm, and quality; respiratory rate and character; skin, lips and nail-bed color. Blood pressure may be measured with conventional sphygmomanometer or an automated ultrasonic device (e.g., Doppler).

A precordial stethoscope is a comprehensive, convenient, unobtrusive, yet cost-effective monitoring device. It allows the listener to monitor heart rate, respiratory rate, and breath sounds concomitantly. Sounds associated with developing airway obstruction may be readily detected.

Pulse oximetry which measures oxygen saturation (Spo_2) is a standard of practice with procedural sedation. It provides early warning of oxygen desaturation before clinical signs develop. Use of pulse oximetry is especially valuable in a patient with a pacemaker to confirm a pulse association with each electrical impulse (Sweitzer, 1998). However, pulse oximetry may not be reliable with extreme oxygen desaturation; marked hypotension;

TABLE 4-4: EXAMPLES OF EMERGENCY EQUIPMENT FOR SEDATION AND ANALGESIA

Appropriate emergency equipment should be available whenever sedative or analgesic drugs capable of causing cardiorespiratory depression are administered. The lists below should be used as a guide, which should be modified depending on the individual practice circumstances. Items in brackets are recommended when infants or children are sedated.

Intravenous equipment
- Gloves
- Tourniquets
- Alcohol wipes
- Sterile gauze pads
- Intravenous catheters [24-22-gauge]
- Intravenous tubing [pediatric "microdrip" (60 drops/ml)]
- Intravenous fluid
- Assorted needles for drug aspiration, intramuscular injection [intraosseous bone marrow needle]
- Appropriately sized syringes [1-ml syringes]
- Tape

Basic airway management equipment
- Source of compressed oxygen (tank with regulator or pipeline supply with flowmeter)
- Source of suction
- Suction catheters [pediatric suction catheters]
- Yankauer-type suction
- Face masks [infant/child]
- Self-inflating breathing bag-valve set [pediatric]
- Oral and nasal airways [infant/child-sized]
- Lubricant

Advanced airway management equipment (for practitioners with intubation skills)
- Laryngeal mask airways [pediatric]
- Laryngoscope handles (tested)
- Laryngoscope blades [pediatric]
- Endotracheal tubes
  - Cuffed: 6.0, 7.0, or 8.0 mm ID
  - [Uncuffed: 2.5, 3.0, 3.5, 4.0, 4.5, 5.0, 5.5, or 6.0 mm ID]
- Stylet (appropriately sized for endotracheal tubes)

Pharmacologic antagonists
- Naloxone
- Flumazenil

Emergency medications
- Epinephrine
- Ephedrine
- Vasopressin
- Atropine
- Nitroglycerin (tablets or spray)
- Amiodarone
- Lidocaine
- Glucose, 50% [10% or 25%]
- Diphenhydramine
- Hydrocortisone, methylprednisolone, or dexamethasone
- Diazepam or midazolam

Note. From "Practice Guidelines for Sedation and Analgesia by Non-Anesthesiologists, An Updated Report by the American Society of Anesthesiologists Task Force on Sedation and Analgesia by Non-Anesthesiologists," 2002, *Anesthesiology, 96*: 1004-17. Retrieved November 26, 2008, from http://www.asahq.org/publicationsAndServices/sedation1017.pdf. Reprinted with permission.

vasoconstriction, as may occur with vasopressors or hypothermia; use of electrocautery; excessive patient movement; and use of certain colors of nail polish, ambient light, or injected dyes that might cause interference.

When respiratory excursions cannot be visually monitored, the use of capnography to measure carbon dioxide (CO_2) in the exhaled breath (end-tidal CO_2 [$ETCO_2$]) is a useful precaution. Because capnography indirectly measures the alveolar air exchange by way of exhaled carbon dioxide, it is capable of detecting hypoventilation not yet detected by pulse oximetry. Clinical signs of hypoxia, such as cyanosis may not be evident until the oximetry reading is below 80% (Riley, 2003).

Ventilation and oxygenation are related processes, but pulse oximetry does not measure ventilatory adequacy. Only direct observation, auscultation, or capnography are suitable monitors of ventilation (Shankar & Deshpande, 2005). During sedation/analgesia administration, electrocardiograph monitoring should be used for all patients with significant cardiac disease and during procedures in which dysrhythmias may be expected, according to the ASA. All equipment should be checked to make sure that alarms are turned on (ASA, 2002).

CNS evaluation requires the attention and analytical skills of the nurse monitor. Excessive CNS depression may be discerned by failure to respond to verbal or tactile stimulation. It may be due to drug overdosage, drug interaction, or respiratory depression resulting in hypoxia or hypercarbia. Although rare, CNS pathology may have occurred.

Agitation and confusion may be due to CNS stimulation. Such stimulation may occur as a result of drugs administered (such as propofol or ketamine), local anesthetic toxicity, hypoxia, or pain. Obviously, a detailed preprocedural history that addresses alcohol or drug abuse or contributory organic conditions will be important in evaluating the cause of CNS symptoms. Proper treatment depends on identifying the cause.

The adverse effect of patient exposure in cool operating rooms is well established, so the patient should be protected as much as possible. For most procedures done in ambulatory surgical settings, the greatest heat loss occurs prior to incision; however, if shivering occurs during the procedure, oxygen consumption increases, which may lead to myocardial ischemia, hypoxemia, and discomfort for the patient. Continuous temperature monitoring devices are usually uncomfortable for the procedurally sedated patient. Axillary temperature monitoring may be the least bothersome method.

Although the patient should be safely yet comfortably positioned to facilitate the procedure before the start of sedation, a comfortable position for the awake patient may become problematic with inactivity and drug-induced interference with muscle tone. Possible pressure areas should be checked periodically to avoid injury. Also check for arms that may have relaxed and slipped putting traction on the brachial plexus.

Positioning is very important for obese patients and those with identified or possibly undiagnosed obstructive sleep apnea. The suggested method is to support the upper back and head so that the patient's head is above the horizontal plane of the chest. Done correctly, the sternum would be in line with the external meatus of the ear (Ebert, Shankar, & Haake, 2006).

AIRWAY MANAGEMENT

The goal of sedation is to have a comfortably sedated but minimally depressed patient who is able to maintain a patent airway independently. However, even at an optimal level of sedation, the patient who lapses into sleeplike episodes may experience some degree of airway compromise. In the supine position, as the pharyngeal muscles relax, the base of the tongue tends to fall backward and may occlude the hypopharynx.

Signs of airway obstruction include:

- retraction of the sternum
- increased respiratory effort
- irregular chest movement
- noisy respirations
- absence of breath sounds by auscultation.

Undetected or untreated, respiratory obstruction will lead to hypercarbia and hypoxemia, which may prove fatal.

At optimal levels of sedation, gently turning the head to the side may relieve minimal obstruction. If not, asking a question that requires a verbal response may cause sufficient arousal for the patient to regain airway control. Questioning will be necessary each time a sleeplike state occurs if there is even mild obstruction. A patient sedated enough to snore may tolerate gentle upward pressure on the mandible.

If the patient becomes deeply sedated, hyperextension of the head into the classic "sniffing" position may pull the tongue forward and away from the posterior pharyngeal wall. The chin should be supported so that the mouth is closed. Adults usually have more normal pharyngeal-laryngeal alignment if the head is elevated on a firm support 3 to 4 inches high. Because of their relative head-to-body proportion, children rarely need additional elevation.

The most effective manual alignment and elevation of the tongue is the triple airway maneuver, produced by lifting the mandible forward and upward with the head tilted backward in the sniffing position (head-tilt, chin-lift, jaw-thrust maneuver) (Figure 4-1). Fingertips are positioned at the angle of the lower jaw and along the ridge, but not into the soft tissue under the jaw. When the tongue and soft tissues have been successfully lifted away from the posterior wall of the pharynx and ventilation is unobstructed, a face mask for oxygen delivery can be held with the thumb and forefinger while three fingers elevate the jaw, thus freeing the other hand for positive pressure assistance. For the novice, two hands may be necessary to control the mask and jaw, so an assistant should be available as needed.

FIGURE 4-1: TRIPLE AIRWAY MANEUVER

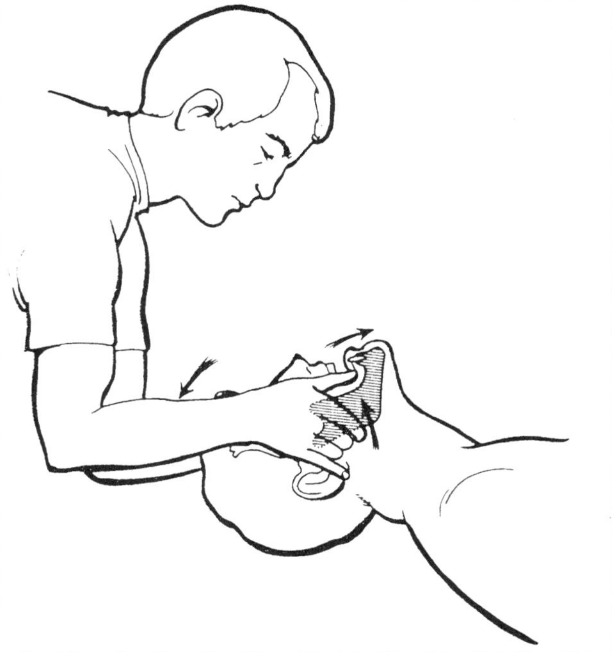

Note. From Emergency Medical Services, U.S. Department of Transportation.

If these techniques fail to establish and maintain a patent airway and adequate ventilation, the deeply sedated patient may tolerate the insertion of a nasal airway. An unconscious patient will tolerate an oral airway if the gag reflex has been obtunded. Retching and vomiting may occur if the reflex is still intact.

Nasal Airway

A nasopharyngeal (nasal) airway is inserted through a nostril into the pharynx behind the tongue, creating a passage to the lower airway for ventilation. A nasal airway does not stimulate the gag reflex, but a traumatic insertion may cause bleeding with accumulation of blood in the oropharynx, which in turn may result in aspiration, laryngospasm, or bronchospasm. Consequently, the use of a nasal airway is contraindicated for patients on anticoagulation therapy or those with septal deformity or nasal polyps.

The nasal airway must be long enough to slip behind the tongue and create a passage between the tongue and the pharyngeal wall. Approximate length may be measured from the patient's nasal entrance to the tip of the earlobe (Kost, 2004). Patency of the nostril should be inspected before insertion is attempted, and the circumference of the tube portion must be less than the size of the naris. The airway must be malleable and well lubricated with water-soluble lubricant before insertion is attempted. Stiff, hard airways should not be used. Gentle insertion may be aided by slightly rotating the airway, but a nasal airway should never be forced. If resistance is encountered in the nasal passage, insertion should be abandoned in that nostril to avoid injury and bleeding.

malleable - pliable

Oral Airway

The oropharyngeal airway is curved to fit over the back of the tongue and hold it away from the posterior pharynx (Figure 4-2). In addition to retching, which may result in hypertension and tachycardia, attempted insertion of an oral airway may cause bradycardia due to vagal stimulation, dental damage, oral lacerations, or laryngospasm.

Using a tongue blade in one hand, the base of the tongue is lifted away from the posterior pharynx as the airway is inserted between the teeth with the curve of the airway conforming to the anatomy of the mouth. If the patient reacts to the tongue blade, insertion of the airway should not be attempted. Appropriate airway size is important; if it is too short, the tongue will not be effectively lifted, and if it is too long, excessive reflex stimulation or trauma may occur. After proper insertion is verified, the nurse should check to make sure the lips or tongue are not caught between the airway and teeth.

An alternate technique for the insertion of an oral airway, often used in emergency situations when a tongue blade is not available, involves inserting the airway in the reverse position (concave portion facing upward toward the operator), then rotating the airway into anatomical position when the tip reaches the back of the tongue. With this method, care must be taken not to push the tongue backward into the pharynx while the airway is being inserted.

In a deeply sedated unconscious patient, if none of these maneuvers resolve the respiratory obstruction, the insertion of a laryngeal mask airway (LMA) or endotracheal tube by an anesthesia provider may be necessary. A properly placed

FIGURE 4-2: INSERTION OF AN OROPHARYNGEAL AIRWAY

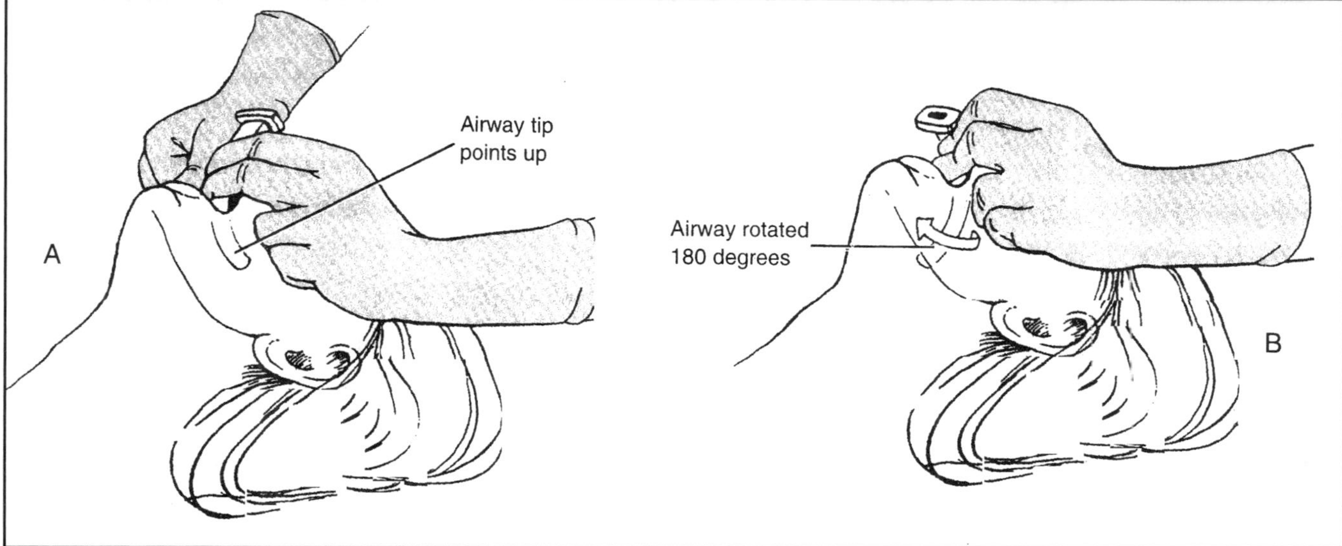

LMA allows positive-pressure ventilation of the lungs for short periods if the peak airway pressure does not exceed 15 cm H_2O (Stone & Gal, 2005), but does not prevent aspiration. An endotracheal tube with a properly inflated cuff seals the trachea, which prevents aspiration and permits control of ventilation for sustained durations. Neither of these two techniques should be attempted without advanced training.

Laryngospasm

Stridor (crowing sounds) or total airway obstruction characterized by rocking abdominal respirations may indicate laryngospasm. Laryngospasm, or spasm of the laryngeal muscles, may be caused by reflex stimulation; airway manipulation; or direct irritation from blood, mucus, or saliva. The vocal cords may be paralyzed in a partially open position, which causes the crowing sounds, or completely closed, preventing ventilation. Positive-pressure ventilation with 100% oxygen is administered in an attempt to stop the spasm, but a small dose of a muscle relaxant, usually the rapid-acting, depolarizing agent succinylcholine, may be needed to relax the laryngeal muscles. Endotracheal intubation may also be necessary.

The nurse monitor should be knowledgeable about and skilled in airway management. An assistant should be readily available at all times during the course of sedation, and an anesthesia provider or person skilled in endotracheal intubation should be called as soon as basic interventions appear to be unsuccessful.

DOCUMENTATION

Meticulous, accurate, and complete documentation during procedural sedation is essential (Riley, 2003). For medicolegal reasons, reference for future procedures for the patient, and quality assurance studies, all facets of the sedation process should be documented and made a part of the patients medical record. Preferably, there should be a dedicated form for sedation.

At a minimum, documentation should include pertinent information from the preoperative assessment, evidence of physical examination, last food intake, and a signed consent for sedation/analgesia administration. Baseline vital signs and patient responsiveness should be noted before administration of any medication.

During the procedure, vital signs should be taken every 5 minutes and recorded. Depending on the monitoring equipment used, some information may be documented automatically, but manual recording ensures that the person caring for the patient is aware of changes in patient status in a timely manner (ASA, 2002).

Medications administered should be documented by dose, route, and time. Total amount and type of IV fluids received, including blood and blood products, should be listed. All nursing interventions and the patient's response should be recorded, as well as significant untoward reactions and their treatments.

Postoperative documentation should provide evidence of monitoring at regular intervals during recovery and list monitoring devices and equipment used. The time of discharge, patient's condition, discharge plan, and the name of the responsible person accompanying the patient should be recorded. Attaching a copy of the patients discharge instructions to the medical record is advisable.

Care should be taken to use institution-approved abbreviations. The next caregiver must be able to correctly decipher these abbreviations. Standard abbreviations are also important if, years later, the nurse is asked to explain the documentation to a lay jury. Legally, errors in charting should not be obliterated; a line through the incorrect statement followed by the correct information is sufficient (Ireland, 1997).

For information not charted at the correct time, a notation of missed entry should be made followed by the information and time of occurrence. This correction is expected to be done in a timely manner, not days or weeks later. Altering or making an addition at that late date constitutes tampering. In many states, tampering with a permanent record is considered a felony (Ireland, 1997).

AORN guidelines expect documentation of patient care during procedural sedation/analgesia to be consistent with recommended practices for documentation of perioperative nursing care.

RECOVERY

After sedation, the patient should be monitored by a nurse or other designated trained personnel until established discharge criteria have been achieved. Level of consciousness and vital signs should be documented at regular intervals. As with all phases of procedural sedation, appropriate monitoring and resuscitation equipment should be immediately available.

Without the stimulation experienced during the procedure, respiratory depression may manifest. Also, if reversal agents were used near the end of the procedure, resedation may occur after reversal effects have subsided. Rate and depth of respiration should be carefully evaluated, and the patient should be encouraged to take deep breaths intermittently. (Recovery and discharge are more fully discussed in Chapter 5.)

DISCHARGE

The patient ready for discharge should be alert, oriented, and demonstrate the preprocedural level of cognition. In addition, as AORN and American Society of PeriAnesthesia Nurses (ASPAN) guidelines state, discharge criteria should require evidence that the patient has returned to a safe physiologic state. Such evidence would include intact protective reflexes; return of motor and sensory control; adequate ventilation; stable vital signs, including temperature; absence of protracted nausea; and absence of significant pain. The surgery site and dressing should be satisfactory.

A patient who has received reversal agents, such as flumazenil or naloxone, should not be discharged before 2 hours have elapsed after the administration of the last drug dose, despite the fact that all other discharge criteria may have been met. Resedation is possible for at least 2 hours following administration of reversal agents. These agents may have shorter effective durations than the medication they were intended to offset (ASA, 2006; White & Recart-Frier, 2005; Shankar & Deshplane, 2005).

A responsible adult must accompany the patient home and remain with the patient at least several hours, preferably overnight, to monitor the extended postoperative period. Written and verbal instructions should be given. It is important that the responsible caregiver, as well as the adult patient, verbally demonstrate an understanding of these instructions because medications used for sedation may affect the patient's recall ability. Additionally, the patient and accompanying adult should understand that driving, as well as operating machinery or using equipment, is not advisable for at least 24 hours after procedural sedation (Riley, 2003).

Parents of small children should be clearly alerted to the possibility that the airway may be dangerously compromised if the head slumps forward when a child is secured in a car seat. Pediatric patients who have received sedation are at significant risk for developing airway-related complications postoperatively because of delayed absorption, lack of stimulation, and less vigilant monitoring (Shankar & Deshplane, 2005) Thus, discharge to home should not be rushed after pediatric sedation.

Any additional discharge requirements that have been established by the ambulatory surgery facility should also be met. Ambulatory surgical or diagnostic facilities should have written recovery and discharge criteria and protocols specifically addressing patients who have received procedural sedation (Riley, 2003).

SUMMARY

The use of sedation has been associated with serious complications and deaths. Institutions that have few complications during sedation attribute this success to:

- proper patient selection
- proper patient preparation
- careful titration of drugs administered
- adequate local anesthesia
- intraoperative monitoring
- supplemental oxygen administration
- maintenance of verbal contact.

Optimal patient care results from the knowledge, vigilance, and experience of the sedation provider (Sweitzer, 1998).

EXAM QUESTIONS

CHAPTER 4
Questions 40-55

Note: Choose the option that BEST answers each question.

40. The term procedural sedation/analgesia implies that the patient
    a. loses sensory discrimination.
    b. responds to verbal communication.
    c. loses airway control.
    d. responds only to reflex stimulation.

41. An inherent danger of deep sedation is
    a. reflex bradycardia.
    b. loss of airway control.
    c. postoperative vomiting.
    d. extrapyramidal stimulation.

42. After a large total dose of diazepam (Valium), impaired coordination may last for
    a. 4 hours.
    b. 6 hours.
    c. 8 hours.
    d. 10 hours.

43. Compared to diazepam, midazolam (Versed)
    a. causes venous irritation.
    b. is longer acting.
    c. produces more effective amnesia.
    d. produces moderate analgesia.

44. Fentanyl (Sublimaze) is considered suitable for moderate sedation/analgesia because of its
    a. lack of respiratory depression.
    b. rapid plasma clearance.
    c. antiemetic properties.
    d. minimal potency.

45. Which of the following opioids is the most potent?
    a. Fentanyl
    b. Alfentanil (Alfenta)
    c. Sufentanil (Sufenta)
    d. Remifentanil (Ultiva)

46. Withdrawal symptoms may be triggered in patients with a history of drug abuse with the use of
    a. long-acting opioids.
    b. agonist-antagonist opioids.
    c. short-acting opioids.
    d. synthetic opioids.

47. A drug that must be available wherever opioids are administered is
    a. flumazenil (Romazicon).
    b. neostigmine (Prostigmin).
    c. naloxone (Narcan).
    d. hydroxyzine (Vistaril).

48. Flumazenil reverses the effects of
    a. barbiturates.
    b. butyrophenones.
    c. phenothiazines.
    d. benzodiazepines.

pg67

49. The administration of small, incremental doses of medication is known as
    a. variable rate infusion.
    b. bolus technique.
    c. titration to effect.
    d. sedative steal.

pg68

50. Fixed dosage combinations of sedatives and analgesics given simultaneously may
    a. decrease total drug dosage.
    b. decrease total cost.
    c. increase time to effect.
    d. increase adverse effects.

pg68

51. Baseline vital signs and patient responsiveness should be documented before
    a. attaching monitoring equipment.
    b. any medication is administered.
    c. the consent form is signed. The allergy band is placed on the patient
    d. the caregiver leaves.

pg70

52. Vasoconstriction, such as that which occurs with perioperative hypothermia, may interfere with accurate
    a. electrocardiography.
    b. pulse oximetry.
    c. capnography.
    d. oscilloscope tracings.

pg72

53. Which device is the most likely to cause bleeding, even when properly sized and inserted?
    a. Nasopharyngeal airway
    b. Oropharyngeal airway
    c. Laryngeal mask airway
    d. Endotracheal tube

pg74

54. Which device protects the airway or lungs from aspiration?
    a. Cuffed endotracheal tube
    b. Nasopharyngeal airway
    c. Oropharyngeal airway
    d. Laryngeal mask airway

pg75

55. A patient who has received moderate sedation/analgesia should be discharged
    a. into the care of a responsible adult.
    b. as soon as reversal agents are effective.
    c. as soon as there is no evidence of orthostatic hypotension.
    d. only after a release has been signed.

pg76

CHAPTER 5

RECOVERY AND DISCHARGE

CHAPTER OBJECTIVE

Upon completion of this chapter, the reader will be able to identify the various aspects of nursing care needed for the safe transition of the patient from the immediate postoperative recovery phase to discharge from the facility.

LEARNING OBJECTIVES

After studying the material in this chapter, the reader will be able to

1. identify essential postoperative patient assessment parameters.
2. identify complications that may occur during recovery from surgery and anesthesia.
3. implement nursing care that will encourage uncomplicated patient recovery.
4. describe the process of discharging a patient from the ambulatory facility.

INTRODUCTION

With the use of short-acting opioids and anesthetics, ambulatory surgical patients are typically alert and in stable condition at the completion of the procedure. The current trend is to separate the postanesthesia care unit (PACU) into Phase I and Phase II recovery stages or to use step-down recovery areas where the patient sits in a reclining chair and, in some cases, may be attended by his or her family or caregiver in preparation for discharge. Advocates believe this arrangement enhances patient and caregiver learning for the extended recovery period and decreases the time to home readiness.

Postoperative care in outpatient settings emphasizes control of nausea and vomiting and adequate pain management to achieve home readiness as quickly as possible. However, ambulatory surgical patients are at risk for postoperative complications as are inpatients undergoing similar procedures; consequently, ambulatory patients require the same level of skilled postoperative care and monitoring. The postoperative period is characterized by a relatively high incidence of potentially life-threatening respiratory and circulatory complications. Patients should be monitored during recovery after all types of sedation or anesthesia, including local infiltration.

As longer and more complex surgical procedures are done on an outpatient basis on patients in less optimal states of health, the issue of adequate postoperative home care must be addressed. The importance of ambulatory surgical facilities developing protocols for quality post procedural care is emphasized.

POSTPROCEDURE CARE

Individual ambulatory care facilities should establish postoperative and PACU policies. Bypassing the PACU and transferring appropriate patients directly to a less intense postoperative recovery area (fast-tracking) may result in significant cost benefits and enhance patient satisfaction. Patients recovering from relatively minor procedures tend to be more satisfied with their postoperative experience if they are separated from those recovering from major procedures. These recovery areas are referred to as Phase II, step-down, sit-up, or progressive care units, and may provide amenities such as recliners, television, music, and light nourishment. They may also function as the discharge area.

Another recovery method, rapid PACU progression (RPP) involves rapid assessment and progression of the patient through the Phase I PACU, with the patient being advanced to the Phase II PACU as soon as Phase I discharge criteria are met, which may be within 15 to 20 minutes rather than the traditional hour. Successful RPP requires collaboration between perianesthesia nursing staff and anesthesia providers, and depends to a considerable degree on motivated and proactive nurses who deliver nursing care efficiently (Mamaril, 2000). Phase I bypass and RPP require close attention and monitoring to ensure that quality of care is not compromised.

Patients undergoing superficial procedures under local infiltration or peripheral regional anesthetics may be able to bypass the PACU and recover in a less intensive area, even if they have been mildly sedated. In some cases, healthy patients undergoing more extensive procedures, (e.g., herniorrhaphy, arthroscopy, minor joint procedures) under a local anesthetic or plexus blockade, might also be admitted to a less intensive recovery unit (Mecca & Serrins, 1997). The decision should be made in consideration of the alternative unit's capacity to deal with analgesic needs and possible surgical or anesthetic complications.

The use of the less soluble volatile anesthetics, such as desflurane (Suprane) or sevoflurane (Sevorane), for maintenance of anesthesia has been shown to result in a large percentage of patients even more eligible for fast-tracking than with propofol (Diprivan) (White & Recart-Friere, 2005; Morgan, Mikhail, & Murray, 2006). An awake, alert patient with no airway difficulties, stable cardiovascular and respiratory functions, and appropriate oxygen saturation may be considered to have acceptable clinical criteria to bypass the PACU and be sent directly to the Phase II setting (Pandit, 1999). However, pre-existing conditions, such as sleep apnea or comorbidities of some elderly patients, may eliminate fast-tracking as an option. Decisions about the necessary level of care for these patients should be made case by case based on the patient's complete health profile and the potential for complications requiring intervention.

Fast-tracking children minimizes parent-child separation, reduces anxiety, and generally improves parental satisfaction with the ambulatory surgical experience. However, the younger the child, the more quickly the postoperative condition may become unstable. When appropriate, ASA grade I or II children who are older than the age of seven, whose surgery has been less than 90 minutes, may be candidates to bypass the PACU and go directly to Phase II (Barnes & O'Brien, 2002).

The American Society of PeriAnesthesia Nurses (ASPAN) holds the position that fast-tracking should involve a collaborative plan of care between the anesthesiology department and perianesthesia service that consists of written guidelines, including those on patient selection, preoperative education of the patient and family, assessment criteria used to evaluate patient readiness to bypass Phase 1 at the end of the surgical procedure, and discharge criteria. In addition, ASPAN asserts that management of the ambulatory facility needs to develop a multidisciplinary, collaborative plan to assure safe and appropriate care when fast-tracking is practiced (ASPAN, 1999). For PACU Phase I bypass the patient must meet all Phase I discharge criteria in the operating room before being transferred to the Phase II recovery area. Patients admitted to the Phase II PACU should not need continuous monitoring or aggressive pain management (Mamaril, 2000). The focus of Phase II care is short-term, nonacute care, such as the 15 to 30 minutes necessary to accomplish final discharge preparation.

The concept of fast-tracking should be explained to the patient and family before surgery, and the family is expected to remain at the facility because the patient should be ready for discharge 30 to 60 minutes postoperatively (Watkins & White, 2001). In appropriate cases, a family member may be with the patient during recovery.

There are minimal levels of care and observation that are widely recognized. In the immediate recovery phase, monitoring and emergency equipment must be readily available. Each patient must have a source of oxygen and suction dedicated to his or her use. Pulse oximetry and blood pressure monitoring are considered to be standards of care, and electrocardiograph monitoring is recommended. Standard emergency equipment and personnel trained to use it are essential.

Admission to the PACU involves the transfer of immediate responsibility for the patient's safety and welfare from the intraoperative anesthesia or sedation provider to the PACU specialist. The patient's name, type of surgery, and pertinent medical history should be described. The nurse should be given a brief summary of the anesthetic technique, course of the operation, total amount and type of fluid administration, complications and the treatment provided, patient's condition prior to transfer, and suggestions for personalized postoperative management, if indicated.

Before accepting responsibility for the patient, the nurse should assess airway patency and then determine and record respiratory rate and character; pulse rate, rhythm, and amplitude; and systemic blood pressure. Level of consciousness and skin color should also be assessed and recorded. Assessment of these conditions every 5 minutes for the first 15 minutes and every 15 minutes thereafter is the generally accepted protocol during an uncomplicated recovery. Recording the patient's temperature may be appropriate on arrival and prior to discharge. Timely and clear documentation of assessment, care, and events in the PACU is important for continuity of care, quality assurance, and medicolegal reasons (Nettina, 2006; McEwen, 2003).

When fast-tracking is not appropriate, families are increasingly being admitted to the PACU. Primary concerns for nurses in these circumstances are personal confidentiality for all patients in the PACU, pain and comfort management, and potential emergency situations. However, ASPAN supports Phase I visitation if guidelines have been developed collaboratively by the perianesthesia and management (ASPAN, 2003).

Nausea and Vomiting

Nausea, vomiting, and pain are the most common management problems in the ambulatory PACU. Along with postoperative bleeding, these factors are the most common causes of hospital admission (Hickok & Weintraub, 1997; Long, 1997; Morgan, Mikhail, & Murray, 2006). The strain of retching and vomiting may also create a risk of postoperative bleeding or hematoma formation.

More than one third of ambulatory surgical patients experience postoperative nausea and vomiting (PONV) (Fetzer, S.A., Hand, M., Bouchard, P.A., Smith, H.H., & Jenkins, M.B, 2005). However, the routine use of antiemetics preoperatively for these patients is controversial because the drugs commonly used have sedative or dysphoric side effects. Metoclopramide and ondansetron have minimal sedative effects. Ondansetron is the most effective agent, whether given preoperatively, intraoperatively, or at the end of the procedure. However, because of cost constraints, ondansetron is commonly reserved for cases in which there is a high probability of nausea and vomiting or the patient experiences protracted PONV.

Considering that prevention is preferable to treatment, a multimodal approach to treating PONV may be appropriate using a combination of medications; for example, a 5-HT_3 receptor antagonist, such as ondansetron, along with low-dose droperidol and dexamethasone (Pasero & Belden, 2006). Also, the postoperative ambulatory surgical nurse should provide the patient with alternative self-care strategies for dealing with PONV that might develop post-discharge (Fetzer et al., 2005). Ambulatory surgical patients are known to develop a high degree of PONV after discharge (Coll, Ameen, & Mosely, 2004).

PONV is usually due to multiple factors, including a high level of anxiety preoperatively (Juarez et al., 2005). Most ambulatory surgical patients do not report retching, so the Rhodes Index of Nausea and Vomiting, a three dimensional scale widely used to assess nausea and vomiting due to chemotherapy or pregnancy is unable to classify the underlying causes of PONV (Coll et al., 2004).

Pain is an often overlooked cause of nausea and vomiting, and sudden movements or position changes should be avoided because opioids may sensitize the vestibule of the ear to motion-induced nausea and vomiting (Hickok & Weintraub, 1997). The incidence of nausea and vomiting is also affected by patient factors, anesthetic techniques, and type of surgical procedure.

Patient Factors

Young patients and female patients, especially if menstruating or in the first trimester of pregnancy, are at the highest risk of developing PONV. Patients with a history of motion sickness or previous postoperative vomiting are at risk, as are those with decreased gastric emptying (e.g., obesity and pregnancy) (Juarez et al., 2005; Tarrac, 2006).

Anesthetic Factors

Opioids are strongly associated with nausea and vomiting, as are certain inhalation anesthetics. Balanced anesthesia, in which opioids are the primary agents, has a high incidence of PONV. Hypotension secondary to spinal or epidural techniques may be a precipitating factor. The IV induction agent propofol causes a low incidence of nausea and vomiting and may have antiemetic properties. Conversely, etomidate for anesthetic induction has a high incidence of postoperative vomiting.

Surgical Factors

Strabismus surgery is commonly associated with nausea and vomiting during recovery, as is orchiopexy. Middle ear surgery is also associated with PONV (Tarrac, 2006). Nose and throat surgery can cause nausea and vomiting in children, who tend to swallow blood and mucus rather than expectorate them. Intra-abdominal procedures are associated with more nausea and vomiting than other procedures, but the highest incidence of PONV in adults is found with laparoscopic procedures. Laparoscopic ovum retrieval procedures are associated with a 54% incidence, whereas other laparoscopic procedures in females are associated with a 35% rate of PONV (Hickok & Weintraub, 1997). Evidence-based clinical practice guidelines for the prevention or management of PONV and postdischarge nausea and vomiting have been developed by ASPAN and are available on their Web site, http://www.aspan.org.

Pain Management

As patients arrive in the PACU more alert and clearheaded, they are also more aware of pain. Relieving postoperative pain with minimal side effects from the analgesics administered is a primary concern in the PACU. Beyond patient comfort, relief of pain reduces sympathetic nervous system response to the pain, thus helping to control hypertension, tachycardia, and agitation. A patient's interpretation of pain sometimes correlates poorly with sympathetic response. The patient may exhibit severe hypertension, tachycardia, and possibly dysrhythmias with minimal complaint of discomfort. Conversely, others may complain of severe pain without clinical signs. This divergence may be related to psychological, cultural, or cardiovascular variations among individuals. Pain management needs to be tailored for different age-groups and various cultural groups (Yellen, 2003).

The current trend is to attempt to qualify perceived pain by using subjective, patient-based scoring systems. These include the visual analog scale (VAS) that ranges from no pain to the worst pain (Figure 5-1); a numerical rating scale where 0 represents the least pain and 10 the worst (Figure 5-2); a numerical descriptor scale with 1 representing mild pain, 2 distressing pain, 3 severe pain, 4 horrible pain, and 5 excruciating pain; and an observational behavior faces scale (e.g., smiling faces or frowning faces) (Figure 5-3). Only the observational behavior faces scale is appropriate for use with a patient who is unable to communicate or cooperate in the assess-

FIGURE 5-1: VISUAL ANALOG SCALE

No Pain ______________________________ Worst Pain

Directions: Ask the patient to indicate on the line where the pain is in relation to the two extremes. Qualification is only approximate; for example, a midpoint mark would indicate that the pain is approximately half of the worst possible pain.

FIGURE 5-2: 0-10 NUMERIC RATING SCALE

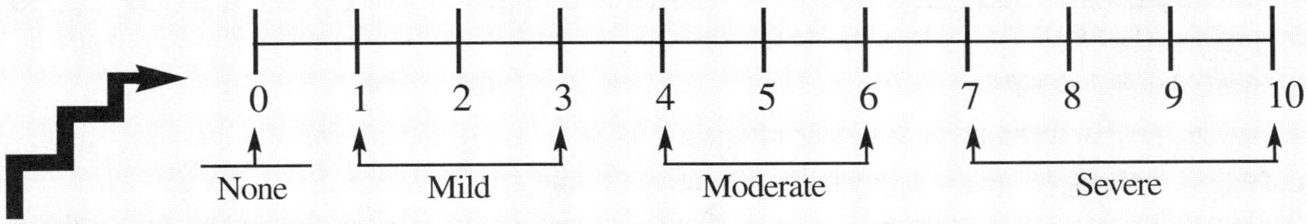

Indications: Adults and children (> 9 years old) in all patient care settings who are able to use numbers to rate the intensity of their pain.

Instructions:

1. The patient is asked any one of the following questions:
   - What number would you give your pain right now?
   - What number on a 0 to 10 scale would you give your pain when it is the worst that it gets and when it is the best that it gets?
   - At what number is the pain at an acceptable level for you?
2. When the explanation suggested in #1 above is not sufficient for the patient, it is sometimes helpful to further explain or conceptualize the Numeric Rating Scale in the following manner:
   - 0 = No pain
   - 1-3 = Mild pain (nagging, annoying, interfering little with activities of daily living [ADLs])
   - 4-6 = Moderate pain (interferes significantly with ADLs)
   - 7-10 = Severe pain (disabling; unable to perform ADLs)
3. The interdisciplinary team in collaboration with the patient/family (if appropriate), can determine appropriate interventions in response to numeric pain ratings.

(McCaffery & Beebe, 1993)

FIGURE 5-3: WONG-BAKER FACES RATING SCALE

TRANSLATIONS OF WONG-BAKER FACES PAIN RATING SCALE*

0–5 coding	0	1	2	3	4	5
0-10 coding	0	2	4	6	8	10
ENGLISH	No hurt	Hurts little bit	Hurts little more	Hurts even more	Hurts whole lot	Hurts worst

Brief word instructions: Point to each face using the words to describe the pain intensity. Ask the child to choose face that best describes own pain and record the appropriate number.

Original instructions: Explain to the person that each face is for a person who feels happy because he has no pain (hurt) or sad because he has some or a lot of pain. **Face 0** is very happy because he doesn't hurt at all. **Face 1** hurts just a little bit. **Face 2** hurts a little more. **Face 3** hurts even more. **Face 4** hurts a whole lot. **Face 5** hurts as much as you can imagine, although you don't have to be crying to feel this bad. Ask the person to choose the face that best describes how he is feeling.

Rating scale is recommended for persons age 3 years and older.

Note. From Hockenberry, M.J., Wilson, D., Winkelstein, M.L., *Wong's Essentials of Pediatric Nursing,* ed. 7, St Louis, 2005, p. 1259. Used with permission. Copyright, Mosby.

Available at http://www.mosbysdrugconsult.com/WOW/facesReproductions.html

ment process (Krechel, 1997), as may be the case with children or geriatric patients.

The reliability of these attempts to quantify pain may be poor because of the great variability among individuals. Scales are most useful when used for gauging response to therapeutic intervention (Mecca & Serrins, 1997). Additionally, although a VAS score of 2 or 3 may signify a comfort level that the patient finds satisfactory at rest, the same score may prove inadequate during coughing, deep breathing, or moving. Comparison of VAS scores both at rest and when ambulating may be more indicative of the adequacy of analgesia as well as home readiness. Current management is directed toward pre-emptive or early treatment that decreases the total required amount of analgesia, which avoids contributing to nausea and vomiting or sedation that may prolong the PACU stay. Preemptive treatment involves the administration of an analgesic of suitable duration of action before the procedure, at the start of the procedure, or during the procedure to provide a smooth, comfortable recovery.

Long-acting opioids, such as morphine or meperidine, are poor choices for ambulatory patients. Conversely, alfentanil and remifentanil are too short acting to provide analgesia of adequate duration, and sufentanil's potency raises safety concerns. Fentanyl, administered by the intravenous (IV) route in small, incremental doses, may be the best choice of opioid analgesic in the ambulatory PACU (Hickok & Weintraub, 1997). IV administration is more flexible and predictable than intramuscular injection.

If IV fentanyl does not provide adequate pain relief, hydromorphone (Dilaudid) given IV or IM has been shown to provide good analgesia with a minimum of nausea and vomiting (Connor & Fogg, 1999). However, hydromorphone is more potent than morphine, has a more narrow range of safety (toxic to therapeutic ratio), and may be associated with a greater risk of respiratory depression (Mulroy & Owens, 1997). Some studies suggest that adverse effects, such as light-headedness, dizziness, sedation, nausea, vomiting, and sweating, are more likely to occur in ambulatory patients. These may be alleviated if the patient lies down. Small doses of a phenothiazine may relieve nausea and vomiting.

Opioid agonists-antagonists, such as nalbuphine (Nubain) or butorphanol (Stadol), tend to produce less respiratory depression but may have a so-called ceiling effect in which increasing doses beyond a certain level may not increase the effect. Intended for flexibility in dosing to meet the unique analgesic needs of each patient, range orders for opiates often result in poor pain management (Gordon et al., 2005). To be effective and safe, range orders should be carefully prescribed and delineated. Since 2004, The Joint Commission requires all organizations to have a policy, based on law and regulation, on the requirements elements for all medication orders. Just as importantly, range orders must be skillfully and carefully interpreted by the perianesthesia nurse. This means the nurse should be familiar with the pharmacokinetics of the medication including: expected time of onset, time to peak effect, duration of action, and possible side effects (Gordon et al., 2005).

Nonsteroidal anti-inflammatory drugs (NSAIDs) do not have the undesirable side effects associated with opioids (e.g., sedation, respiratory depression, nausea and vomiting, urinary retention), and they may be continued after discharge. They may act synergistically with opioids without causing respiratory depression (Chung & Lam, 1997). Combining NSAIDs with morphine may result in a 30% to 50% morphine-sparing effect while significantly lowering the incidence of nausea, vomiting, and sedation (Kamming, Chung, Williams, McGrath, & Bruna, 2004; Ebert, Shankar, & Haake, 2006). To be effective immediately postoperatively, NSAIDs may be given orally 1 hour before anesthetic induction or IM after induction. Oral ibuprofen has been reported to be more effective than fentanyl for postoperative analgesia in patients undergoing laparoscopic surgery (Hickok & Weintraub, 1997). Multimodal analgesia using acetaminophen, NSAIDs, and morphine has been found to be as effective as intraperitoneal injection of a local anesthetic and/or morphine (Keita, Benifla, Le Bouar, & Porcher, 2003).

Ketorolac (Toradol), a parenteral NSAID, may be given IV or IM. Its potency is believed to be similar to that of morphine, but for severe pain, supplementation with small doses of an opioid may be necessary. Some surgeons may be concerned that ketorolac may cause bleeding at the surgical site because of inhibitory action on platelets; therefore, the use of ketorolac should always be confirmed with the surgeon (Connor & Fogg, 1999). Ketorolac is 50 times more potent than naproxen (Ebert, Shanker, & Haake, 2006). Because nonselective NSAIDs, such as ibuprofen and naproxen, may increase bleeding time they are usually discontinued before surgery (Pasero & Belden, 2006)

Like aspirin, all NSAIDs may interfere with platelet aggregation (Chung & Lam, 1997), and they are usually contraindicated in patients at risk for gastrointestinal (GI) or surgical bleeding or those receiving anticoagulant therapy. The operative site of any patient receiving NSAIDs should be closely monitored for any sign of bleeding or hematoma formation. The risk of operative site bleeding or GI bleeding is increased with doses higher than 120 mg daily when used for more than 5 days and in older patients. A study of patients who underwent lumbar laminectomy and were treated with NSAIDs found a detrimental effect on bone union when high doses of 120 mg to 240 mg per day were given for 5 days (Ebert, Shanker, & Haake, 2006). Interference with osteoclast activity affecting bone healing is a concern for orthopedic surgery (Brislin & Rose, 2006).

Significant renal disease is also a contraindication to the use of NSAIDs. Because of the decrease in renal function associated with age, the dosage of NSAIDs should be reduced in elderly patients. When the patient is able to take oral medication, acetaminophen, acetaminophen with oxycodone, or ibuprofen are frequently prescribed for transition to discharge.

Acetaminophen is the most commonly used oral analgesic worldwide because it is effective for mild pain and has few adverse effects when the recommended daily dose is not exceeded. The maximum adult oral dose is 4 g (4,000 mg) over 24 hours (Kamming et al., 2004). Acetaminophen has a significant opioid-sparing effect, and it can be administered rectally to children. Unlike NSAIDs, it does not irritate gastric mucosa, affect platelet function, or cause renal dysfunction. Acetaminophen may be combined with any analgesic to increase pain relief (Pasero & Belden, 2006).

Providing postoperative pain relief for obese and morbidly obese patients without causing excess sedation and concomitant respiratory depression may be challenging; however it is necessary to avoid upper airway obstruction caused by excess pharyngeal tissue. In obese patients, even brief periods of obstruction or hypoventilation may cause a precipitous drop in arterial oxygen saturation due to reduced functional residual capacity and increased oxygen need (Ebert, Shanker, & Haake, 2006).

Similarly, respiratory depression resulting from pain management medications must be avoided in patients with obstructive sleep apnea (OSA). If the use of an opioid becomes necessary, opioid antagonists should be immediately available. Procedures involving the upper airway and areas near the diaphragm have been found to result in more complications in patients with OSA (Moos & Cuddeford, 2006).

Multimodal therapy using combinations of analgesics that act by different mechanisms may result in additive effects. Lower doses of each analgesic used in combination reduce the possibility of adverse effects (Kamming et al., 2004). Using a multimodal approach, analgesic therapy may provide a continuum of care from surgery through at home recovery (Joshi & Kehlet, 2006). An example of multimodal therapy is to combine an opioid, NSAID, acetaminophen, and local anesthetic; each acting on different types of pain transmission.

Combination techniques may include the use of NSAIDs with alpha$_2$-adrenergic receptor agonists, such as clonidine, or NMDA receptor agonists, such as ketamine. Clonidine has hypnotic, sedative, sympatholytic, and analgesic properties. Ketamine enhances the analgesic effects of morphine by inhibiting the action of NMDA receptors. Although not commonly used in the ambulatory surgery setting, a single dose of 0.1 mg to 0.15 mg per kg given at the end of surgery may produce long-lasting analgesia without the adverse effects of dissociation and hallucination. The effect may be due to spinal cord protection from centrally mediated hyperalgia as a consequence of the peripheral noxious stimulation from surgery (Kamming et al., 2004). An atypical opioid that is structurally related to codeine, tramadol has fewer side effects, but is 10 to 15 times less potent than morphine. Because tramadol has been associated with seizures on rare occasions, it is contraindicated in patients with a history of seizures, in those who are on medications that lower the seizure threshold, and in patients with head trauma (Brislin & Rose, 2006)

Pain is a potent stimulus that may support respiration, alertness, and blood pressure. Consequently, when pain is relieved, hypoventilation, somnolence, or hypotension may develop. Hypovolemic patients may exhibit precipitous hypotension when sympathetic support due to the stimulation of pain ceases, resulting in venous and arterial vasodilation. Hypotension and vasodilation may be made worse by histamine release secondary to opioid administration (Mecca & Serrins,

1997). Additionally, the depressant effects of analgesics may cause hypoventilation that may result in hypoxemia and respiratory acidosis. Patients who are confused and agitated due to hypoxemia, acidosis, or cerebral ischemia may be difficult to differentiate from those with true pain, but it is essential that no further analgesic is administered until these causes have been eliminated.

Local anesthetic infiltration of the incision, or anesthetic splashed into the wound near the end of the procedure, provide effective postoperative analgesia (refer to Chapter 3). Nerve blocks are also effective but carry the risk of injury due to lack of sensation and motor control, especially if an extremity is involved. Intra-articular boluses of local anesthetic, with or without morphine, reduce the need for supplementary analgesia after orthopedic surgery.

As ambulatory surgery continues to evolve, alternative routes of analgesic administration, such as the use of nasal sprays, are being used and evaluated. Opinion is strongly divided on patient-controlled analgesia (PCA) using IV opioids. Some investigators feel it is absolutely contraindicated, whereas others believe it reduces the total amount of drug required and may be advantageous for early discharge.

Insufficient pain relief may be the cause of various complications. Hypertension and tachycardia in response to pain may lead to myocardial ischemia and heart failure; splinting of abdominal or chest wounds may lead to hypoventilation, atelectasis, and pneumonia; and there is evidence that neurohumoral responses to pain can interfere with wound healing (Chung & Lam, 1997).

In ambulatory surgery, poor pain management may delay discharge and also cause patient dissatisfaction with the entire surgical experience. Because effective pain management is a vital component of patient care, The Joint Commission developed pain management standards that are mandatory for all health care organizations to comply with for accreditation. The Joint Commission's first evidence-based standards, were developed from sources such as the American Pain Society and the Agency for Healthcare Research and Quality (Gordon et al., 2005).

Common Postoperative Complications

Respiratory problems are the most frequently encountered complications in the PACU, with the majority due to airway obstruction, hypoventilation, or hypoxemia. Such problems, if undetected or untreated, may result in serious morbidity or mortality. Routine monitoring of pulse oximetry in the PACU leads to earlier detection and fewer adverse outcomes. However, despite advances in medications and techniques, the rate of complications is similar to those in 1990 (Tarrac, 2006).

Airway Obstruction

Obstruction of the airway is most frequently associated with patients who are still semiconscious, especially those in supine or sitting positions. Unless contraindicated by the surgery, laying the patient on his or her side creates less chance of airway obstruction. This positioning is especially important for patients with OSA not using continuous positive airway pressure (Moos & Cuddelford, 2006). The lateral position also promotes drainage of respiratory secretions. This position is particularly applicable for pediatric patients in whom laryngospasm is more likely to occur if secretions or blood collect near the glottis and irritate the vocal cords.

Patients who have undergone surgery of the nasal passages, mouth, throat, or neck have the potential for serious compromise of the airway. Airway or respiratory problems may develop over several hours postoperatively, so prolonged postoperative observation is required when airway compromise is possible (Conahan & Young, 1997).

Hypoventilation

Residual sedative, narcotic, or anesthetic effect, residual neuromuscular paralysis, and airway obstruction are the most frequent causes of postoperative hypoventilation. Benzodiazepine effects may respond to reversal with flumazenil, and narcotic effects may be reversed with naloxone. However, ambulatory surgical patients should not be discharged until at least 2 hours after the last dose of a reversal agent was administered because of the possibility that resedation may occur (ASA, 2002; Kost, 2004; White & Recart-Frier, 2005; Shankar & Deshpande, 2005).

Although patients with OSA are at increased risk for hypoventilation, with the exception of emergency situations, supplemental oxygen should be used cautiously because it may reduce hypoxic drive resulting in increased incidence and duration of apneic episodes (Joshi, 2006). Even with the use of pulse oximetry, oxygen supplementation during recovery may hamper the detection of hypoventilation or atelectasis (Moos & Cuddeford, 2006).

Although the availability and use of shorter-acting nondepolarizing neuromuscular blocking agents (NMBAs) has reduced the incidence of residual paralysis, it still occurs and may be fatal if not recognized and treated. The characteristic sign presented by a patient in the PACU is shallow, labored respiration (Brown, M., 1997). Asking the patient to lift his or her head off the support and hold that position for 5 seconds provides some indication of motor ability. Testing with a peripheral nerve stimulator is more definitive.

When the core body temperature or acid-base balance is not normal, the metabolism of neuromuscular agents may be affected, Patients who appear to be breathing well when admitted to the PACU may later develop signs of inadequate respiration. If conscious, the patient may complain of respiratory distress or have difficulty speaking, but unconscious patients may drift into hypoventilation (Kervin, 2002).

Oxygen and manual or mechanical respiratory support must be given immediately when residual paralysis is present. Nondepolarizing NMBAs may be reversed with an appropriate reversal agent, but a phase II block following the depolarizing muscle relaxant succinylcholine is pharmacologically more complex to treat. In either case, ventilation must be assisted until adequate spontaneous respiration resumes. If the patient is unconscious, intubation may be necessary.

Hypoxemia

Causes of hypoxemia include hypoventilation, airway obstruction, and ventilation-perfusion abnormalities, aspiration, or pulmonary edema. Cyanosis is a late sign of hypoxemia and may not be seen in patients with low hemoglobin or hematocrit levels. To avoid irreversible cellular damage or a fatal outcome, oxygen supplementation and ventilatory support must be provided while the cause of the hypoxemia is established and treated.

Hypotension

The most common cause of hypotension in the PACU is hypovolemia (Cowling & Haas, 2002). Hypotension is usually due to either decreased venous return to the heart or left ventricular dysfunction (Morgan, Mikhail & Murray, 2006). Blood loss and inadequate fluid replacement resulting in hypovolemia reduce the venous return to the heart. A significant drop in blood pressure, accompanied by an increase or decrease in heart rate, may indicate hemorrhage, circulatory failure, or fluid shifts (Shumaker, 1997). Hypotension due to developing hemorrhagic shock is usually accompanied by tachycardia; cold, moist, pale, or cyanotic skin; and increased restlessness or agitation, often described as air hunger. Initial treatment includes administering oxygen and, unless contraindicated, increasing IV fluid flow rate and elevating the legs.

Sympathetic blockade due to residual spinal or epidural anesthesia, opioid effect, or allergic reactions are also possible causes of hypotension. Patients on steroids may be developing an addisonian crisis. The possibility of blood transfusion reaction must also be considered. Oxygen supplementation should be provided while the cause is identified and treated. Dizziness associated with sitting up (orthostatic hypotension) or dangling legs suggests incomplete recovery of sympathetic function (Knoerl, McNulty, Estes, & Conley, 2001).

Hypertension

Postoperative hypertension is frequently seen in patients with hypertensive disease and systemic atherosclerosis. More common causes are pain, bladder distention, hypercapnia, hypoxemia, or fluid overload. Tachycardia and arteriosclerosis may promote an exaggerated response to stimuli that may result in vasoconstriction (Tarrac, 2006).

Uncontrolled hypertension may lead to cerebral hemorrhage or myocardial ischemia (Chung & Lam, 1997). The underlying cause of hypertension must be identified and treated. Perioperative cardiovascular complications are becoming more common in the ambulatory surgical setting as older and less healthy patients are managed as outpatients (Conahan & Young, 1997).

Tachycardia

Although some types of surgery, such as thyroidectomy, are more likely to produce tachycardia during recovery, more common causes include pain, hypovolemia, hypoxia, hypercapnia, anemia, and fever. In addition to the operative site, pain may be caused by an overdistended bladder or even a strain resulting from positioning during the procedure (Tarrac, 2006). Treatment of tachycardia should be aggressive to assure adequate coronary output and peripheral perfusion. Depending on the cause, treatment may consist of volume expansion for hypovolemia, analgesics for pain, or medication to produce beta blockade.

Shivering

Shivering may be due to hypothermia that develops intraoperatively and is also associated with emergence from volatile anesthetics. Sepsis, allergy, and transfusion reaction may also be serious causes. Intense shivering increases oxygen consumption and physiologic stress that may be detrimental to patients with cardiovascular or pulmonary impairment. Oxygen administration is appropriate. Inadequate pain control is another possible cause. If the shivering does not respond to external warmth, such as warm blankets, small doses of IV meperidine are usually effective.

Shivering is uncomfortable for the patient and may itself increase wound pain, and increase intraocular and intracranial pressures. Clonidine, doxapram, or alfentanil are other medication options that should not delay discharge from an ambulatory facility (Belani, 2005).

Agitation and Delirium

Agitation is usually due to inadequately controlled pain, but fear and discomfort from bladder or gastric distention are also possible precipitating factors. Ketamine, large doses of phenothiazines (particularly in geriatric patients), and anticholinergics (e.g., atropine, scopolamine) (especially in children) may produce agitation and delirium. Patients recovering from ketamine benefit from a quiet atmosphere with subdued lighting; IV diazepam may also be beneficial. IV physostigmine is often effective for delirium associated with phenothiazines and anticholinergics.

More serious causes of agitation and delirium include surgical complications, such as intra-abdominal hemorrhage, hypoxemia, acidosis, or hypotension (Morgan, Mikhail & Murray, 2006). Restlessness and excitement due to alcohol or drug withdrawal in the unsuspected addict may be extremely difficult to diagnose and treat (Chung & Lam, 1997). However, perianesthesia nurses should always consider that agitation and restlessness may be signs of hypoxia that need careful evaluation (Kervin, 2002).

Somnolence

Prolonged somnolence is most frequently due to residual anesthetic, sedative, or analgesic drug effect. Reversal agents such as naloxone for opioids and flumazenil for benzodiazepines may be effective. However, hypoventilation is commonly the cause of delayed emergence from inhalation anesthetics, so airway patency and other possible causes of hypoventilation should be investigated and relieved before pharmacologic intervention. Prolonged somnolence may also be due to serious intraoperative events (e.g., cerebrovascular accident or systemic disease, such as a patient with diabetes who becomes hypoglycemic).

Dehydration

Unrecognized, untreated dehydration due to nothing-by-mouth status may be responsible for some common postoperative adverse effects. One study suggests that, unless medically contraindicated, the rapid administration of an isotonic electrolyte solution 30 minutes before surgery may significantly reduce some of these effects (Winslow & Jacobson, 1997). Based on the premise that overnight fasting causes a fluid deficit of at least 1 liter in a 70-kg adult, in addition to the normal daily water requirement of approximately 30 ml/kg, the fluid should be administered at 20 ml/kg (Kozar & Moore, 2005).

In the previously mentioned study, patients who received increased IV hydration preoperatively showed significant decreases in dizziness, drowsiness, and thirst at 1/2 hour and 24 hours postoperatively. However, nausea was decreased significantly with preoperative hydration only at 24 hours (<5% vs. >10%), and there was no difference in vomiting, hemodynamic conditions, or time to meet discharge criteria. Optimal hydration during anesthesia was associated with low rates of PONV (Tarrac, 2006)

Less Common Postoperative Complications

Less common, but dangerous postoperative complications include malignant hyperthermia (MH) and postintubation laryngitis. Because MH (refer to Chapter 6) may first occur in the postoperative period, it is important for perioperative nurses to be familiar with signs of a developing episode. Postoperative situations that may present similar or confusing symptoms include mismatched blood transfusions, infectious fever, anticholinergic drug therapy, dehydration, thyroid storm, uncontrolled pain, and overzealous patient warming. However, unexplained tachycardia, tachypnea, dysrhythmia, cola-colored urine, and temperature increase require immediate evaluation (Karlet, 1998).

Postintubation laryngitis may occur after a short-term intubation, or after a long procedure because of irritation from the endotracheal tube. Primarily involving the subglottic area, postintubation laryngitis may cause laryngeal edema and airway obstruction. The most obvious symptom is stridor, but the recovering patient should be monitored for sudden changes in oxygen saturation (preferably by pulse oximetry), decreased breath sounds, and changes in mental status. Initially, treatment consists of supplemental oxygen and cool humidity, but the use of an aerosolized vasoconstrictor (Geiger-Bronsky, 1998) or steroids may become necessary.

Recovery from Regional Anesthesia

Regional anesthesia is not synonymous with lack of possible postoperative complications. For example, the following conditions may develop after regional anesthesia administration:

- Hypotension, accentuated by position changes, is a common problem following spinal and epidural anesthesia due to residual sympathetic blockade. Early head-up positions and ambulation are associated with an increased occurrence of postdural puncture headache after spinal anesthesia.
- An unusual delay in recovery of motor function or sensation following nerve block, spinal, or epidural anesthesia may be a serious complication requiring treatment. Although regional anesthetics are effective, the patient is at risk for injury due to lack of sensation or poor coordination.

- Many patients receive sedation in addition to regional anesthesia and need to be observed in a controlled recovery area until they are alert, stable, and suitable for discharge. Patients who are heavily sedated or hemodynamically unstable following regional anesthesia should receive supplemental oxygen in the PACU (Morgan, Mikhail & Murray, 2006).

Although toxicity related to a local anesthetic may be delayed as much as 1 hour, depending on absorption, it more commonly occurs soon after injection. Consequently, patients who have had their procedures done with local infiltration and no sedation frequently bypass the Phase I (PACU) recovery stage and are prepared for discharge in the Phase II, or step-down, area.

DISCHARGE CRITERIA

Patients who are discharged prematurely are more likely to develop postoperative complications or suffer injury due to psychomotor impairment. Home readiness does not imply that the patient has the ability to make important decisions, to drive, or to return to work. These activities require complete psychomotor recovery, which is often not achieved until 24 to 72 hours after surgery (Morgan, Mikhail, & Murray, 2006).

Numerical scoring systems have been developed that provide objective assessment of the patient's progress and readiness for discharge and serve as medicolegal documentation of the patient's status. The Postanesthesia Discharge Scoring System (PADS or PADSS) is an example of an assessment tool developed specifically for ambulatory patients (as opposed to the older Aldrete scoring system for hospitalized patients, which does not consider level of hydration, pain, or ability to ambulate). Although the Aldrete scoring system was updated in 1995 to include the use of pulse oximetry for oxygen saturation levels in addition to nail and mucous membrane color, it is best used to indicate readiness for transition from Phase I to Phase II recovery (i.e., from the termination of anesthesia until protective reflexes and motor function return) (Kamming & Chung, 2004).

The PADS system assesses vital signs; ambulation and mental status; pain, nausea, and vomiting; surgical bleeding; and intake and output. The maximum score is 10, but patients with a score of 9 or greater are considered suitable for discharge. This system is most appropriately used to track transition from Phase II to Phase III (i.e., when the patient is ready for discharge to home, where late Phase III takes place) (Ead, 2006).

Each ambulatory surgical center should have established evidence-based discharge criteria applicable to all types of patients and procedures. Legally, such criteria should address postanesthesia and postprocedural practice approved by the governing medical body responsible for the facility (Ireland, 1997). In the Standards of Perianesthesia Nursing Practice (2006), the ASPAN requires documented assessment and evaluation of patients at the time of discharge, in compliance with written policy.

Subject to limitations imposed by the surgery, common patient status requirements for discharge include:

- vital signs stable for 30 to 60 minutes
  - blood pressure within 20 mm Hg of the preoperative level
  - stable pulse rate and rhythm, near preoperative levels
  - respirations consistent with preoperative depth and rate with no croupy cough, especially in children
- orientation to person, time, and place
- coordination sufficient to dress self
- adequate mobility (may be influenced by surgery)
  - ability to walk without dizziness with assistance
  - ability to move from wheelchair to car and from car into home safely

- minimal nausea and vomiting
- pain controllable with oral analgesia
- no bleeding at operative site
- no sign of hypothermia or unexplained temperature elevation
- ability to take oral fluids (if specified by physician)
- no signs of hypovolemia
- ability to void (if specified by physician)
- adequate sensory and motor function return to lower limbs following spinal or epidural anesthesia
- consistent signs of progression in return of sensation and motor control in upper limb following peripheral nerve block
- adequate vision.

Opinion differs on requirements for oral intake and voiding. Requiring all patients to void and tolerate oral fluids is believed to cause unnecessary discharge delays. Consequently, voiding and drinking have been removed from the PADS system (Ead, 2006). Although there is concern that the patient be able to tolerate oral fluid intake to prevent dehydration, some believe insisting that patients take oral fluids before they wish to may actually increase the incidence of nausea and vomiting. Similarly it is expected that patients who have received sufficient fluid replacement probably will urinate before meeting all discharge criteria; but if they have not, and they have not undergone surgery that might interfere with urination, some authorities contend that the patients may be released with instructions to call if they have not voided in 6 hours (Kamming & Chung, 2004).

Although patients usually achieve discharge status more rapidly if oral intake and voiding are not part of the discharge criteria, this practice may be questionable for elderly men with a history of urinary problems and for patients who have undergone rectal, genitourinary, or gynecological surgery or inguinal herniorrhaphy. In addition, it is particularly important that the patient be able to void after spinal or epidural anesthesia. The ability to void is a sign of recovery of autonomic function (Chung & Lam, 1997). Postoperative urinary retention may be affected by the agent used to produce the spinal or epidural and any opioid given concomitantly. Hydrophilic opioids, such as morphine, are more likely to cause urinary retention than are lipophilic opioids such as fentanyl (Eads, 2006).

Mobility without dizziness is important for the outpatient. Despite progression to a phase II or step-down area, where the caregiver or a family member may be in attendance, the patient should not be allowed to attempt standing or walking for the first time unless a PACU staff member is assisting. For those who have had spinal or epidural anesthesia, evaluation is recommended to be done in three stages: sitting up only, dangling legs, and standing with assistance.

The postoperative analgesia associated with peripheral nerve blocks reduces the need for pain medication; however, with the absence of sensation or motor control comes the danger of inadvertent injury. The patient must be instructed to protect the limb and monitor circulation, sensation, and swelling. After a brachial plexus block it may be advisable to place the affected arm in a sling for protection. Digits should be evaluated for adequate circulation, and sensation and circulation should be satisfactory in an extremity on which a tourniquet was used during surgery.

Discharge readiness does not equate with street fitness. Safe discharge from the ambulatory facility not only requires the return of vital signs and systemic functions to near preoperative levels, but it also requires the patient to be free from significant cognitive or psychomotor impairment. Residual effect of sedatives and anesthetics may last 24 hours or more, during which time the patient should not engage in activities that require quick reflexes or sound judgment. For the same reason, patients should be cautioned against drinking alcoholic beverages or taking sedatives or antihistamines for 24 hours. When discharged to home, patients with OSA are at increased risk because of the possibility of residual anesthetic or analgesic effect (Moos, Prasch, Cantral, Huls, & Cuddeford, 2005).

A patient who has received pharmacologic reversal agents, such as flumazenil (Romazicon) or naloxone (Narcan), should not be discharged before 2 hours have elapsed since the last administration. Despite the fact that all other discharge criteria have been met, resedation is possible for at least 2 hours after administration of reversal agents.

A responsible adult must accompany the patient home and preferably remain with the patient overnight or longer to monitor the extended recovery period. These arrangements should have been finalized preoperatively. Appropriate family or caregiver support is vital to provide a safe transition from the facility to home (Pasero & Belden, 2006). Written and verbal instructions should be provided. In their 2009 National Patient Safety Goals, The Joint Commission stipulates that a complete list of medications should be provided to the patient on discharge. It is important that the responsible caregiver, as well as the adult patient, verbally demonstrate an understanding of these instructions because residual effects of medications may affect the patient's recall. In addition, the responsible adult should be provided with a 24-hour emergency phone number and be cautioned about what to monitor and what actions to take. Parents of small children should be clearly alerted to the possibility the airway may be dangerously compromised if the head slumps forward when a child is secured in a car seat.

All discharge requirements established by the ambulatory surgical facility should be met, and the patient should have no symptoms that would threaten a safe recovery. If there is any question of fitness for discharge, the nurse should seek a direct evaluation and discharge from the physician. Some facilities require that the anesthesia provider evaluate the patient for discharge.

Despite the proven reliability of scoring systems and guidelines used for discharge, they are just tools that should not replace the critical thinking or professional judgment of the nurse (Ead, 2006). For example, patients with diabetes must be able to take and retain fluids before discharge. Patients with a family history of MH should be monitored for 4 hours prior to discharge (Ead, 2006). Obese and morbidly obese patients require extended monitoring beyond achieving acceptable scoring and guideline standards because of the danger of respiratory obstruction when their pain is controlled (no longer acting as a stimulus).

Similarly, patients suspected of or diagnosed with OSA require longer postoperative monitoring (Bachenberg, 2005) and need to be observed at least 3 hours before discharge because postoperative complications usually occur within 2 hours (Joshi, 2006). These patients should not be discharged until they are able to maintain preoperative oxygen saturation levels when breathing room air (Moos & Cuddelford, 2006). Lastly, when deciding when to discharge the patient from the facility, the nurse must consider the distance of the nearest medical facility from the patient's home.

POSTDISCHARGE FOLLOW-UP

Patients should receive a postdischarge follow-up telephone call the next day to verify safe and uneventful recovery, identify complications, evaluate potential problems, and address any concerns or grievances related to the procedure. Follow-up calls are regarded as a standard of practice. To protect privacy, the Health Insurance Portability and Accountability Act requires that written permission must be obtained to leave postoperative follow-up telephone messages by voice mail or with a designated person (AORN, 2006).

The postdischarge call may be more productive if made in the late afternoon or early evening of the first day after discharge rather than that morning (Dewar, Scott, & Muir, 2004; Horvath, 2003). Usually the morning of the first day postdischarge is less than 24 hours postoperative and the patient may still be benefiting from the analgesic given after the procedure; whereas nearly 50% of patients experience moderate to severe pain after 4 p.m. Pain at this time and on day two postdischarge may be significantly predictive of the length of recovery time until normal activity is possible (Horvath, 2003).

The registered nurse who contacts the patient must be able to communicate appropriately and make valid assessments through telephone contact. A protocol developed by the ambulatory center that provides a checklist of questions reduces the ambiguity of decision-making concerning how to handle a problem (Barnes & O'Brien, 2002). The nurse should have thoroughly reviewed the patient's chart and be able to provide explanations for minor symptoms, give general reassurance, and give appropriate advice on contacting the physician or getting emergency assistance if necessary. The nurse who discharged the patient from the facility is the ideal person to evaluate the patient's status the following day.

Ongoing studies suggest that at least 3 days of successive follow-up phone calls provide important support and guidance on coping with pain (Dewar, Scott, & Muir, 2004). Inadequate pain control may be associated with adverse reactions such as nausea, vomiting, and dizziness, which, as well as pain, may be causes of readmission (Mitchell, 2004). Successive follow-up telephone calls promote better pain management because the nurse may advise the patient about changing the timing and amount of medication, which also tends to reduce possible uncomfortable side effects (Watt-Watson, Chung, Chan, & McGillion, 2004).

Although postoperative pain intensity depends primarily on the type of surgical procedure, a large number of patients experience severe pain that is inadequately controlled during recovery at home; some for as long as 7 days. Laparoscopic sterilization is frequently associated with severe pain for at least 3 days due to ischemia that develops, along with the carbon dioxide gas inflation. By the seventh postoperative day, 30% of these patients still have considerable pain (Coll & Ameen, 2006). Patients undergoing laparoscopic cholecystectomy and vaginal hysterectomy may also be expected to have significant pain for several days. In a 2003 study of the intensity of pain associated with ambulatory procedures, laparoscopic cholecystectomy ranked second after lumbar microdiscectomy (Kammimg et al., 2004).

Shoulder surgery has been found to result in considerably more pain and pain-related recovery interference, such as difficulty sleeping, than hand, knee, or ankle surgeries (Kamming et al., 2004; Watt-Watson, 2004). Varicose vein surgery also is associated with lingering postoperative pain.

To some extent poorly controlled pain during at home recovery may be due to a lack of patient understanding as to how to manage pain, which highlights the need for preoperative and postoperative patient education as to what to expect and how to deal with it (Coll & Ameen, 2006). Patients commonly have biases and misconceptions that affect how compliant they are with taking postoperative pain medication. Some patients fear that taking a drug strong enough to obtund their pain will lead to addiction, whereas others quickly associate pain medication with nausea and vomiting and stop taking the medication. Still others with inadequate relief of pain "double up" on their medication, treating themselves through trial and error, which may result in greater problems (Watt-Watson et al., 2004).

However, the most common reasons for noncompliance are that patients do not remember the instructions they were given verbally at discharge; do not remember they were given written instructions at discharge; or just do not read the printed material they received. For these reasons, it is important that a full account of discharge instructions and materials provided be documented on the patients chart (Dewar, Scott, & Muir, 2004).

DISCHARGE EDUCATION

Although discharge planning and initial postoperative education should begin preoperatively, shortened monitored postoperative recovery times challenge nurses to provide patient education in an environment that may be less than ideal for learning. However, provision of clear, concise discharge instructions is a primary nursing responsibility (McCamant, 2006).

Patients and caregivers may feel unprepared and anxious about the responsibility of postoperative care. Well-informed patients actively involved in their own care have decreased complication rates, increased compliance, reduced recovery time, greater satisfaction, and require less analgesia (Bumgarner & Evans, 1999; Fox, 1998). Studies have shown that patients want very detailed instructions concerning their at-home recovery. (Dewar, Scott, & Muir, 2004).

Patients and caregivers often fear that they will not be able to provide adequate care after discharge. Even worse, they are concerned that they may do the wrong thing and cause harm. The more major the surgery, the greater is their apprehension. During follow-up telephone contact, patients often express their displeasure about being discharged when they did not feel well enough to leave the facility.

Care of the incision is a major concern. Most important is the fear that the incision may open, especially after sutures or staples are removed. Consequently, the nurse should explain the healing process simply and clearly in lay terms. It is reassuring to the patient and caregiver when they understand that within 48 hours after the incision was made the wound has closed (epithelialization) (Fox, 1998).

Ambulatory patients frequently are discharged with a wound dressing in place and are concerned about causing infection when changing or removing the dressing. To allay this fear, the patient (appropriate to age and mental status) and caregiver should be instructed how to do this, preferably with the patient and caregiver giving a return demonstration. If appropriate, viewing the incision with the nurse will facilitate the patient's ability to identify changes such as redness or swelling that should be reported. They should also be alerted that increased pain and fever are other symptoms of possible infection.

Patients usually equate recovery with the absence of pain and the ability to return to normal daily living, but deficits in self-care activities may persist postoperatively for as long as a week. This is common even after herniorrhaphy. Protracted inability to care for oneself may lead to anxiety and frustration (Lupien, Schoneboom, & Wren, 2000). Teaching practical applications of postoperative care, in addition to the customary medical instructions, should be part of postoperative patient education. Concerns that should be addressed include:

- bathing and washing hair
- dietary advice
- prevention of constipation secondary to analgesic medications
- allowed activities
- activities to avoid (lifting, driving, etc.)
- therapeutic rest vs. "taking it easy."

For example, grocery shopping, child care, and doing laundry all fall into the category of lifting. Patients also need to be aware that both pain and medication might contribute to slower reaction times.

After anorectal procedures, patients seem to particularly need reassurance. Consequently, adequate preoperative instruction and postoperative follow-up may reduce their anxiety and assist recovery. Many patients wrongly avoid solid food to avoid bowel movements. These patients need to be specifically advised to drink three to four glasses of water or juice with the prescribed laxative, rather than being told to "drink plenty of fluids." They also need to understand that sitz baths promote healing and are not simply for cleanliness (Dewar, Scott, & Muir, 2004).

Postoperative muscle pain (myalgia) may add to the delay in a return to normalcy. Perioperative factors contributing to postoperative muscle pain include age, gender, medications such as succinylcholine, position during surgery, and abdominal insufflation for laparoscopy. Pain in the back and upper body may be the most incapacitating (Lupien et al., 2000). Treatment is primarily palliative.

Although patients should be instructed to take the prescribed pain medication on a continuous basis for 1 to 2 days, suggesting nonpharmacologic methods of pain management may decrease the total amount of analgesic required and ease the transition from medication. Cognitive-behavioral strategies include relaxation, distraction, imagery, meditation, and prayer. Patients with cognitive deficits tend to benefit from the distraction provided by music, and may also be capable of rhythmic breathing relaxation exercises with coaching from the caregiver. Physical interventions include applications of heat or cold, massage, movement, and rest or immobilization. Applications of heat or cold, if ordered by the physician, alter the pain threshold, reduce muscle spasm, and decrease local swelling. Simple rest is an important part of pain management that should not be overlooked, especially in the first 48 hours postoperatively.

Because of the varied patient population undergoing ambulatory surgery and the strained learning environment, functional literacy, or the ability to apply what is read to everyday life, may be even less than normal. Standard printed postoperative instructions given to the patient on discharge might be improved with images and personalized notations made by the nurse. Procedure specific easy-to-read patient care guides similar to clinical care maps, but using patient-friendly language and images, may be an effective education tool (Bumgarner & Evans, 2000).

In addition to medication/prescriptions, specific instructions given by the surgeon and a 24-hour telephone number should be provided. Patients being discharged from an ambulatory surgery facility are best prepared if the perioperative nursing staff has addressed the practical postoperative self-care topics that the patients and caregiver want to know, as well as the specific postprocedure instructions they need to know.

SUMMARY

Exemplary recovery care and discharge procedures contribute to the low complication rate (less than 2%) associated with ambulatory surgery. Unanticipated admissions for surgical outpatients range from 0.3% to 1.4% (Eads, 2006). Even though the types, duration, and number of ambulatory procedures continue to increase, to maintain and improve these favorable statistics, postoperative ambulatory surgical patient care must not be compromised; rather, evidence-based care will become more of a necessity.

EXAM QUESTIONS

CHAPTER 5
Questions 56-71

Note: Choose the option that BEST answers each question.

56. When receiving a patient into the PACU, the nurse should first assess the patient's
    a. circulation.
    b. awareness.
    c. muscle tone.
    d. airway.

pg83

57. An IV induction agent that may have antiemetic properties is
    a. etomidate (Amidate).
    b. thiopental (Pentothal).
    c. methohexital (Brevital).
    d. propofol (Diprivan).

pg84

58. Which type of medication may sensitize the patient to motion-induced nausea and vomiting?
    a. Anticholinergics
    b. Butyrophenones
    c. Benzodiazepines
    d. Opioids

pg84

59. Balanced anesthesia, in which an opioid is the primary agent, may result in a high postoperative incidence of
    a. hypotension.
    b. nausea and vomiting.
    c. dyspnea.
    d. muscle rigidity.

pg84

60. In children, the surgical procedure most frequently associated with postoperative nausea and vomiting is
    a. strabismus correction.
    b. appendectomy.
    c. inguinal herniorrhaphy.
    d. fracture reduction.

pg84

61. In adults, the highest incidence of nausea and vomiting is associated with
    a. endoscopy.
    b. laparoscopy.
    c. arthroscopy.
    d. fluoroscopy.

pg84

62. For the ambulatory surgical patient, preemptive treatment is advocated for postoperative
    a. allergic reactions.
    b. pain management.
    c. pneumonitis.
    d. seizures.

pg86

63. NSAIDs, such as ibuprofen, are contraindicated for pain management in patients with
    a. insulin-controlled diabetes.
    b. significant renal disease.
    c. chronic obstructive pulmonary disease.
    d. congestive heart failure.

pg88

64. Which drug may act synergistically with opioids without causing respiratory depression?

pg87
a. Midazolam
b. Promethazine
c. Droperidol
(d.) Acetaminophen

65. The most frequently encountered complication in the PACU is

pg89
a. hypertension.
(b.) airway obstruction.
c. shivering.
d. sympathetic blockade.

66. Unless contraindicated by the surgery, the safest position for a child during recovery is

pg89
a. supine.
b. Fowler's.
(c.) lateral.
d. Trendelenburg.

67. The characteristic signs of postoperative residual neuromuscular blockade are

pg90
(a.) shallow, labored respirations.
b. deep, slow respirations.
c. paradoxical respiration.
d. diaphragmatic respiration.

68. The most common cause of postoperative hypotension is

pg90
(a.) hypovolemia.
b. pain.
c. vomiting.
d. hyperthermia.

69. On sitting up or standing for the first time after the procedure, the patient may experience

pg91
a. cardiac dysrhythmia.
(b.) orthostatic hypotension.
c. benign hypertension.
d. transient hyperthermia.

70. A quiet atmosphere with subdued lighting is recommended for a patient recovering from which anesthetic?

pg91
a. Propofol
(b.) Ketamine (Ketalar)
c. Thiopental
d. Halothane (Fluothane)

71. Because of poor motor coordination or lack of sensation, a patient who has had a peripheral nerve block has an increased risk of

pg92
a. hypotension.
b. pain.
(c.) injury.
d. nausea.

CHAPTER 6

COMPLICATIONS AND EMERGENCIES

CHAPTER OBJECTIVE

Upon completion of this chapter, the reader will be able to recognize serious complications and emergencies that may occur during ambulatory surgery and anesthesia.

LEARNING OBJECTIVES

After studying this chapter, the reader will be able to

1. identify serious complications that may occur intraoperatively.
2. discuss implications of delayed recognition of developing complications.
3. select appropriate nursing interventions to enhance favorable treatment outcomes.
4. recognize the need for constant preparedness to effectively treat complications.

INTRODUCTION

As the familiar axiom states, there is no such thing as a minor surgical procedure or minimal anesthesia. Technical developments or patient variables, not always identifiable or controllable preoperatively, may lead to complications or emergencies. Being aware of their possible occurrence and being prepared to quickly and efficiently treat untoward intraoperative events allows the perioperative nurse to play a pivotal role in the successful resolution and positive outcome of these events. Key nursing strategies include being knowledgeable about possible complications or emergencies; making sure the operative area is equipped with appropriate medications and well-maintained emergency equipment; knowing how to use emergency equipment; recognizing early signs of complications or emergencies, and alerting the appropriate members of the operating room team. Anesthesia providers routinely need the cooperation and assistance of the perioperative nurse to facilitate optimal patient care; when emergencies occur, the nurse becomes an invaluable assistant.

Certain surgical procedures are recognized as having the inherent possibility of developing complications, regardless of the operative setting in which they are performed. Several of these procedures, currently and frequently performed in ambulatory surgical facilities, are reviewed in this chapter. As outpatient surgery evolves and expands, so too will the hazards involved.

Interventions initiated by the perioperative nurse should be consistent with the facility's guidelines, the state's nurse practice act, the nurse's level of skill and training, and the actions of a prudent nurse.

SURGICAL COMPLICATIONS

Technical Complications

Complications may occur as a result of inadvertent technical errors. Examples include pneumothorax caused by puncture of the pleura during upper abdominal surgery or laceration of an organ or blood vessel during laparoscopy. Also, when pathology is found to be more advanced than anticipated, a more extensive procedure and postoperative hospital admission may be necessary.

Laparoscopic Surgery

To create a space for visualization, instrumentation, and manipulation within the abdominal cavity, a pneumoperitoneum must be established by instilling gas into the cavity, which lifts the abdominal wall away from the viscera. Carbon dioxide (CO_2) or nitrous oxide (N_2O) may be used, but because nitrous oxide supports combustion, carbon dioxide is usually used. Trocars are inserted through the skin at strategic points in the abdomen and are used to insert and remove instruments, remove fluid, and extract tissue or organs (Wadlund, 2006). Inadvertent error may occur with these necessary steps as well as during the procedure.

Carbon dioxide is rapidly absorbed across the peritoneal membrane into the general circulation resulting in hypercarbia and respiratory acidosis, which requires careful monitoring and treatment (Hunter, 2005) because both conditions may produce myocardial depression. Theoretically, because of the high solubility of carbon dioxide, there would be rapid absorption of an embolus, should one occur. However, if a sufficient quantity is rapidly taken into the circulatory system, an air lock in the right side of the heart may occur (Small, 1998). Injuries to vessels of the abdominal wall are most common with complicated surgeries, especially procedures using lateral trocar placement and larger trocars. Life-threatening hemorrhage may result from injury to the inferior gastric artery (Sutton, Rodgers, Hurd, & Mutone 2005).

The creation of a pneumoperitoneum necessarily results in increased intra-abdominal pressure, but overpressurization may have serious consequences. Intrathoracic space may be reduced leading to inadequate ventilatory exchange and inadequate cardiac output. Pulmonary edema may develop in patients with compromised cardiac effectiveness. Regurgitation and aspiration of gastric contents may be caused by increased pressure on the diaphragm. Excessive pressure may also cause carbon dioxide to diffuse into the bloodstream resulting in hypercarbia and dysrhythmias.

Although postoperative pain in the shoulder and neck due to irritation of the phrenic nerve is common following laparoscopic abdominal surgery, excessive pressure may damage the nerve, as well as cause severe discomfort for the patient. Because the phrenic nerve supplies the diaphragm, respiratory adequacy may also be affected. The use of an insufflator that automatically vents excessive carbon dioxide is the best precaution, but applying pressure to the abdomen to evacuate residual gas before the last trocar is removed at the end of the procedure is also advisable (Rothrock, 2003).

Gas Embolism

With increased intra-abdominal pressure, if a blood vessel is injured, the pressure may allow carbon dioxide to enter the circulation. Inadvertent placement of the carbon dioxide insufflator into a blood vessel or organ is another possible cause of gas embolism.

Symptoms of gas embolism include tachycardia, hypotension, cyanosis, dysrhythmia, and a characteristic "mill wheel" murmur. Evidence of right heart block or strain may be seen on an electrocardiogram if the embolus is large (Wadlund, 2006). Shock and cardiac arrest may develop. End-tidal carbon dioxide ($ETCO_2$) may increase before declining as a result of excretion of carbon dioxide that has been absorbed into the blood (Small, 1998). Sudden development of hypercapnia during intra-abdominal carbon dioxide insufflation means a embolism has developed (Chung & Lam, 1997). Routine analysis of $ETCO_2$ during laparoscopic surgery may detect even small emboli.

Treatment of gas embolism includes:

- administering 100% oxygen
- increasing ventilation to increase carbon dioxide excretion
- placing the patient in the left lateral decubitus head-down position to allow the gas to rise away from the pulmonary circulation
- inserting a multiple-orifice central venous catheter to aspirate gas
- supporting blood pressure with vasopressors and IV fluids
- eliminating source of gas, if possible

(Wadlund, 2006; Hunter, 2005).

If severe hypotension develops, external cardiac massage may be used to fragment large bubbles (Wadlund, 2006; Sutton et al., 2005).

Carbon Dioxide Escape

Carbon dioxide may escape from the abdomen to the pleural spaces, pericardium, mediastinum, or subcutaneous tissues. Clinical signs may range from shock and respiratory failure (due to pneumothorax) to swelling of the face and neck with crepitation, due to gas in the tissues. Head and neck swelling is usually treated conservatively with elevation of the head postoperatively.

Peak inspiration pressures and chest movements should be closely monitored during laparoscopic surgery. A sharp increase in peak inspiratory pressure may indicate tension pneumothorax. Treatment of pneumothorax consists of 100% oxygen with positive end-expiratory pressure (PEEP) (Wadlund, 2006). Chest tube insertion to evacuate the gas may be necessary (Small, 1998).

Laparoscopic Abdominal or Pelvic Surgery

Unrecognized injury to a large blood vessel or the bowel may become life threatening postoperatively. Symptoms of internal bleeding are more readily observable, whereas those of bowel involvement may not be properly identified for as long as 72 hours after surgery (Wadlund, 2006). Therefore, any unusual or persistent postoperative complaint of abdominal discomfort, no matter how vague, should be thoroughly assessed and documented.

Laparoscopic cholecystectomy has been associated with marked deficits in postoperative pulmonary function; the adequacy of respiration and oxygen saturation must be closely monitored. Treatment of nausea and vomiting, which reportedly occurs in 12% to 52% of laparoscopic cholecystectomy patients, is critical because if the factors are not adequately controlled hospital admission may be required (Fleisher et al., 1999). The length of stay for patients who were carefully assessed preoperatively usually ranges from 4 to 8 hours (Lam, Miranda, & Hom, 1997), with 6.6 hours considered average (Fleisher et al., 1999). If discharge criteria are not met within these parameters, hospital admission may need to be evaluated. Time to discharge is comparable to other major surgeries, such a lumbar laminectomy, after which patients usually attain discharge readiness within 4 to 6 hours (Scanlon & Richards, 2004).

Ophthalmic Surgery

Ophthalmic procedures have been the most frequently performed ambulatory surgeries. Adult ophthalmic surgery is most frequently performed using a nerve block with procedural sedation. The following complications apply to extraocular procedures (e.g., strabismus correction, lacrimal duct probing, lid surgery, enucleation) and intraocular procedures (e.g., cataract extraction, vitreoretinal surgery, glaucoma-related procedures):

- Oculocardiac reflex – due to pressure on the eyeball or traction on the eye muscles. Causes sudden, severe bradycardia and possibly asystole. Treatment involves immediately releasing the pressure or traction, administering IV atropine, or if the patient is under general anesthesia, deepening the level of anesthesia. Continuous monitoring of the heart rate during ophthalmic procedures is essential. Establishing and maintaining IV access is advisable.
- Periorbital block complications – possibility of intravascular injection of local anesthetic, globe perforation, and brady dysrhythmias, but have a lower risk of serious complications than retrobulbar blocks (Donlon, Doyle, & Feldman, 2005). Retrobulbar block complications include hematoma or retrobulbar hemorrhage, globe perforation, systemic local anesthetic toxicity, brady dysrhythmias, or central nervous system anesthesia due to subdural spread. These blocks are used for intraocular operations, such as cataract extraction. Topical anesthetic agents are becoming a much more common anesthetic choice for ophthalmic procedures by many physicians.
- Hypoventilation – a sedated patient with his or her face covered by drapes may experience hypoxemia. Pulse oximetry and careful, continuous observation of chest excursion is necessary.
- Coughing or movement – resulting in globe injury or vitreous extrusion.

Otolaryngology and Oral Surgery

Complications following surgery involving the nose, throat, and mouth are frequently associated with postoperative bleeding and swelling, which may compromise the airway and sometimes develop into life-threatening situations. These patients require constant observation during recovery, rapid complication intervention, and judicious discharge. The nurse must always be prepared for emergencies with the otolargyngology patient.

If the procedure has been done under general anesthesia with endotracheal intubation, the endotracheal tube is usually left in place with the cuff inflated until the patient's gag and swallowing reflexes have returned. Careful suctioning of the mouth and pharynx is necessary during recovery and prior to release of the cuff (Morgan, Mikhail, & Murray, 2006).

After dental surgery, patients often have packing in place that may obstruct the airway, especially if the patient is somnolent. Procedures done under local or topical anesthesia may result in systemic local anesthetic toxicity. Topical local anesthesia is rapidly absorbed from mucous membranes. In addition, dental injury is possible due to surgical instrumentation or airway manipulation.

Ear surgery is associated with a high incidence of postoperative nausea, vomiting, dizziness, and vertigo. If an incision was made, bleeding and infection are possibilities.

An environmental complication to be avoided is injury from an unstable microscope used during surgery. The microscope should be equipped with an emergency stop to prevent patient injury.

Cosmetic and Reconstructive Surgery

Despite the fact that many cosmetic procedures are considered office procedures, serious complications are possible.

Lipoplasty is associated with major fluid compartment shifts, resulting in hypotension, electrolyte imbalance, and edema. Large amounts of local anesthetics injected throughout the procedure may cause systemic toxicity. Hidden subdermal bleeding and pulmonary thromboemboli are postoperative complications associated with liposuction (Aker, 2001)

Breast reduction or augmentation may involve significant blood loss and the possibility of pneumothorax from inadvertant injury to the pleura.

Rhinoplasty patients may experience postoperative bleeding and airway compromise. Postoperative bleeding and swelling may distort an incision and affect final results. Postoperative retching or vomiting may cause hematoma or stress a suture line.

Hypoventilation may result when a sedated patient's face is obscured by surgical drapes, leading to hypoxemia. Having one of the patient's hands exposed, using pulse oximetry, and maintaining voice contact, if appropriate, aid monitoring.

Gynecologic Procedures

Laparoscopic and laser surgery techniques have broadened the scope of ambulatory gynecologic procedures that are suitable for the ambulatory setting. Consequently, the following complications associated with gynecologic procedures may be characteristic of these techniques.

- Inadvertent injury to such abdominal structures as the bladder, bowel, and blood vessels during laparoscopy may occur resulting in bleeding or infection.
- Embolism may result secondary to gas infused during hysteroscopy or the creation of the pneumoperitoneum necessary for abdominal laparoscopy.
- Perforation of the uterus may occur during intra-uterine procedures.
- Systemic fluid absorption during intrauterine flushing, as during endometrial ablation, may result in severe electrolyte imbalance and fluid overload.
- Trendelenburg position may compromise ventilation, especially in obese patients.
- Lithotomy position may result in nerve injury affecting the legs if not carefully managed.

Orthopedic Procedures

Since the development of the arthroscope, many orthopedic procedures that formerly required hospitalization for surgical exposure of the joint (i.e., arthrotomy) are now being done as ambulatory procedures. Immediate and delayed potential complications of arthrosopic surgery include:

- bleeding into the joint
- systemic local anesthetic toxicity
- infection
- neurovascular injury secondary to the use of a pneumatic tourniquet.

Thyroid Surgery

The development of minimally invasive surgical approaches and ultrasonic technology for intraoperative bleeding control have made it possible to perform thyroid surgery in the ambulatory setting for carefully selected, otherwise healthy individuals.

However, the major complications associated with thyroid surgery remain:

- injury to the laryngeal nerve
- hemorrhage
- upper airway injury
- hypocalcemia.

Laryngeal nerve damage affecting the vocal cords is assessed as soon as the patient is able to speak, and upper airway injury may be expected to manifest soon after extubation. However, hemorrhage remains a concern during recovery and requires careful monitoring. The prophylactic use of oral calcium supplementation reduces the possibility of life-threatening hypocalcemia (Terris, Moister, Seybt, Gourin, & Chin, 2006).

Urologic Procedures

Endoscopic procedures account for a large number of ambulatory urologic procedures. Associated complications include:

- systemic absorption of irrigating fluids, resulting in serious electrolyte imbalance, including hyponatremia
- hemorrhage; infection; and injury to bladder, ureters, or urethra.

Volume Depletion

Volume depletion may result from extensive blood loss during surgery or inadequate fluid replacement. Postoperative bleeding may require a return to surgery. Such bleeding may be readily observable, as with a hematoma forming in the area of operation or a tonsillectomy patient coughing up blood. Any hematoma that expands rapidly and/or results in hypotension, tachycardia, or overlying tissue ischemia requires prompt surgical exploration (Brown, O.W., 1997). Covert bleeding may be identifiable only by characteristic signs of impending hemorrhagic shock, including hypotension, tachycardia, pallor or cyanosis, oliguria, or restlessness and apprehension.

ANESTHETIC COMPLICATIONS

Aspiration

Aspiration of gastric contents is a potentially fatal complication of anesthesia (Chung & Lam, 1997). When gastric contents are regurgitated into the hypopharynx and then inhaled into the lungs, consequences include bronchospasm, pneumonitis, or atelectasis.

Aspiration is a potential problem in deeply sedated and anesthetized patients who are unable to maintain a patent airway and have obtunded gag and cough reflexes, which prevent clearing the airway. Although aspiration of blood or other foreign material may seriously interfere with oxygenation, aspiration of strongly acidic gastric fluid is corrosively damaging as well. As little as 25 ml of gastric fluid with a pH of 2.5 may result in severe pneumonitis. Aspirated solids obstruct the tracheobronchial tree, resulting in atelectasis, and may require bronchoscopy for evacuation.

Clinical signs of atelectasis are usually immediately apparent, whereas signs of acid pneumonitis may not occur for several hours. Signs of pneumonitis may include cyanosis, tachycardia, tachypnea, rales, and rhonchi (Nettina, 2006). Severe cases may develop into pulmonary edema with hypoxemia. For mild cases, treatment is largely supportive to ensure adequate oxygenation. The effectiveness of steroid therapy is controversial, but antibiotics may be necessary to control secondary infections (Chung & Lam, 1997). Massive aspiration may require controlled ventilation and PEEP to provide adequate arterial oxygenation.

Patients at the greatest risk for perioperative aspiration include those with a hiatal hernia; gastroesophageal reflux disease; increased intra-abdominal pressure, such as morbid obesity and pregnancy; bowel obstruction; noncompliance with nothing-by-mouth status; and emergency circumstances (White & Recart-Friere, 2005; Riley, 2003). Endotracheal intubation after rapid-sequence anesthetic induction is usually indicated for these patients. Postoperatively, extubation or deflation of the cuff is not advisable until consciousness and laryngeal reflexes have returned (Morgan, Mikhail, & Murrat, 2006; Stone & Gal, 2005).

Prophylactic Medications

The following medications are used prophylactically to lessen the possibility of aspiration.

- Histamine-2 (H_2)-receptor antagonists, such as cimetidine (Tagamet), ranitidine (Zantac), or famotidine (Pepcid), may be given IV, but usually they are given orally the evening before surgery and 1 to 2 hours before induction to inhibit gastric acid secretion. H_2-receptor antagonists only affect the pH of gastric acids secreted after administration.
- Metoclopramide (Reglan) orally 1 to 2 hours or IV 45 minutes before induction accelerates gastric emptying.
- Nonparticulate antacids, such as Bicitra or Polycitra, neutralize acidity. Given orally, 30 minutes before surgery or induction, they do increase gastric volume but are less damaging

to the alveoli than particulate antacids, such as magnesium hydroxide.

Sellick's Maneuver

In situations where the possibility of regurgitation is increased, the nurse may be asked to apply pressure to the cricoid cartilage (i.e., perform Sellick's maneuver) from the start of induction until the endotracheal tube cuff is inflated and proper placement is verified.

Finger pressure over the cricoid cartilage, below the thyroid notch and cricothyroid space, compresses the esophagus against the sixth cervical vertebra, decreasing the mechanical possibility of regurgitation of gastric contents into the hypopharynx.

Cricothyrotomy

In the event that adequate ventilation cannot be achieved and tracheal intubation is technically impossible due to conditions such as anatomic malformation, scarring over the neck, previous radiation of the neck, or cervical spine restrictions, cricothyrotomy (cricothyroidotomy) may be necessary. A large-gauge catheter or special cannula is inserted into the cricothyroid membrane. Whereas a cannula, such as the Nu-Trake, is large enough to permit adequate ventilation and positive-pressure inflation, a 12- or 14-gauge catheter requires a pressure of 50 psi to generate sufficient gas flow (transtracheal jet inflation) (Morgan, Mikhail, & Murray, 2006). Tracheostomy may be done after the patient is adequately oxygenated.

Malignant Hyperthermia

Malignant hyperthermia (MH) is a hypermetabolic, hyperthermic syndrome that develops in genetically predisposed individuals when exposed to volatile inhalation anesthetics or the depolarizing muscle relaxant succinylcholine. The term malignant refers to the seemingly uncontrollable hyperthermia, which had a mortality rate of 70% to 80% when the syndrome was first identified in the 1960s. Advances since then have reduced the mortality rate to approximately 10%, but a successful outcome depends on early recognition and aggressive treatment. It is not associated with carcinoma.

MH occurs most commonly in older children and young adults, especially males. Many people with the inherited predisposition also exhibit other skeletal muscle abnormalities, such as strabismus, inguinal hernia, clubfoot, cardiomyopathy, or excessive muscular bulkiness (Chung & Lam, 1997). These individuals tend to be prone to joint dislocations and are frequently intolerant to caffeine-containing foods.

Some muscle diseases have been associated with a high incidence of MH or MH-like occurrences, including Duchenne's muscular dystrophy, myotonia, osteogenesis imperfecta, central core disease, congenital muscular dystrophy, and King-Denborough syndrome. Even patients with less common myopathies may demonstrate MH-like episodes that respond to treatment with dantrolene (Dantrium), that occur during general anesthesia without the use of potent inhalation agents or succinylcholine (Brandom, 2005). Because MH does not develop with every anesthetic exposure, susceptible individuals may have no family history (Rosenberg & Rothstein, 2006).

Since the genetic defect associated with porcine MH was identified more than 10 years ago, more than 100 human families have been identified as MH susceptible (Brandom, 2005). Although an elevated serum creatine kinase level implies susceptibility in individuals with a known family history, the only definitive test involves muscle biopsy and contracture testing that is only performed at a relatively small number of centers worldwide (Brandom, 2005; Morgan, Mikhail, & Murray, 2006). Because contracture testing can only be done on individuals at least 10 years old and weighing more than 40 kg, genetic testing may become especially important in establishing a diagnosis in children with a family history suggestive of MH (Brandom, 2005).

MH is thought to be initiated by loss of control over calcium ion sequestration and reuptake in skeletal muscle fibers, leading to contracture, increased oxygen consumption, and increased production of heat and lactate (Chung & Lam, 1997). Symptoms may occur immediately after minimal exposure to a triggering agent or later in the PACU. Episodes have been known to recur within 24 hours after the initial attack subsided (Morgan, Mikhail, & Murray, 2006).

Early signs of hypermetabolism resemble a light level of anesthesia and are characterized by increased carbon dioxide production, tachycardia, tachypnea, and increased cardiac output. However, these signs quickly develop into anaerobic metabolism, metabolic acidosis, cellular hypoxia, muscle cell necrosis, hyperkalemia, myoglobinemia followed by disseminated intravascular coagulation, renal and cardiac failure, and coma (Chung & Lam, 1997; Murphy, 1997).

Rigidity of the masseter muscles of the jaw (i.e., trismus) after receiving succinylcholine during halothane anesthesia may be one of the first signs of imminent MH, especially in children. However, rigidity also occurs in 1% of normal children. Because inappropriate hypercapnia and hypoxemia are early signs, the capnograph and pulse oximetry recordings have been recognized as the best form of monitoring to give early warning of an impending crisis (Chung & Lam, 1997). Temperature may rise as much as 1°C every 5 minutes after the attack is established; however, fever is a late and inconsistent sign of hypermetabolism, so routine temperature monitoring is of little value for very brief anesthetics, but it is necessary for operations lasting more than a few minutes (Murphy, 1997). The Malignant Hyperthermia Association of the United States (MHAUS) advises that temperature should be monitored in all but extremely brief procedures (Rosenberg & Rothstein, 2006).

Immediate treatment of MH consists of:

- discontinuing known anesthetic triggering agents
- hyperventilating the patient with 100% oxygen at a high flow rate
- concluding surgery as quickly as possible
- administering IV dantrolene
- cooling the patient if his or her temperature is above 38°C; cooling measures include:
  - applying ice packs to the body surface
  - applying iced irrigating solutions to the stomach, bladder, and open body cavities as necessary to maintain the patient's temperature below 40°C
  - administering iced IV fluids
  - providing heat exchange with a pump-oxygenator.

Central venous access, arterial cannulation for blood samples, core temperature probe, and indwelling urinary catheterization must be established. Intubation is necessary for airway control and hyperventilation. Sodium bicarbonate is given to treat acidosis and hyperkalemia, and mannitol or furosemide (Lasix) may be indicated for diuresis to avoid renal failure caused by the end products of cell degeneration.

To deal with the multifaceted treatment of MH, additional skilled personnel will be needed immediately. The reconstitution of dantrolene is a time-consuming process that requires the concerted efforts of more than one person to complete the task as quickly as possible. All perioperative nursing personnel should be familiar with this procedure.

Research has shown that warming the sterile water used to reconstitute the dantrolene to 41°C can reduce the usual 2 minutes per bottle preparation time by at least 30 seconds. Because seconds count when treating MH, this time saving can be significant (Baker & Landriscina, 2007).

An adequate supply of dantrolene (at least 36, 20-mg vials), refrigerated IV solutions, ice, and other appropriate supplies should always be immediately available wherever general anesthesia is administered, including in office-based settings (Morgan, Mikhail, & Murray, 2006; Rosenberg & Rothstein, 2006).

If the surgery cannot be completed immediately, anesthesia must be maintained by IV agents. Barbiturates, opioids, propofol, etomidate, droperidol, and nondepolarizing muscle relaxants are considered safe for the MH patient. Phenothiazines are controversial because they may increase intracellular calcium (Murphy, 1997).

Dantrolene, which blocks calcium release, is the mainstay of treatment. Elevated temperature should drop as the drug takes effect. The drug is administered IV incrementally to effect. For example, 2 mg/kg of dantrolene may be given every 5 minutes to a total dose of 10 mg/kg if needed, although higher total doses have been used when necessary (Gronert, Pessah, Muldoon, & Taute, 2005). An alternative treatment uses an initial-dose of dantrolene 2.5 mg/kg repeated IV every 5 minutes until the crisis is resolved (Morgan, Mikhail, & Murray, 2006). Because MH may recur several hours after the first attack and the half-life of dantrolene is approximately 6 hours, a sustaining dose of 1 mg/kg may be given IV every 6 hours for 24 to 48 hours (Morgan, Mikhail, & Murray, 2006).

Although dantrolene is the only specific drug for treatment of MH and must be used, patients receiving calcium channel blockers, such as verapamil, may suffer from serious cardiac depression and dangerously high levels of potassium from the drug combination. For the same reasons, calcium channel blockers are contraindicated in the treatment of the tachycardia and dysrhythmias that may occur with MH (Dorian, 2005). Theophylline, aminophylline, epinephrine, or digoxin may intensify an MH attack (Nettina, 2006).

Emergency consultation is available 24 hours a day at 1-800-644-9737 (1-800-MH-HYPER), the hotline provided by the MHAUS. Instructions for therapy should be kept with the supplies, and every ambulatory facility, including office-based settings, should have established guidelines for preoperative management of the MH-susceptible patient so that all precautions are taken to avoid a life-threatening crisis. All personnel should be prepared to safely treat an MH crisis. The anesthesia department should be notified as soon as the procedure is scheduled. Because of the intensity involved in treating an occurrence, mock departmental drills are recommended. MHAUS explains these procedures in manuals for hospitals, ambulatory surgery centers, and offices doing outpatient surgery (Rosenberg & Rothstein, 2006).

Individuals with confirmed MH are advised to wear medical alert identification (ID). They and their first-degree relatives should register with the North American Malignant Hyperthermia Registry. A variety of educational materials are available for medical professionals and MH-susceptible individuals and their families from MHAUS by phone (800) 98-MHAUS, fax (607) 674-7910, or the Web at http://www.mhaus.org. The organization also sponsors a medical ID program.

ALLERGIC REACTIONS

Anaphylactic and Anaphylactoid Reactions

Atopy - refers to the genetic tendency to develop allergic diseases.

Individuals with a history of atopy, including bronchial asthma, hay fever, eczema, and food allergies, may be more likely to experience a reaction to an IV drug because of a genetic predisposition that causes the production of increased amounts of immunoglobin E (IgE) antibodies (Vitkun, 1997).

Anaphylactic reactions (e.g., anaphylaxis, anaphylactic shock) and anaphylactoid reactions may cause life-threatening situations; the mechanisms differ, but clinical signs are similar and death may occur due to respiratory failure or circulatory collapse. Initially, these reactions may be extremely difficult to recognize in a patient under heavy sedation or general anesthesia because symptoms are similar to those seen with many other situations associated with surgery and anesthesia. However, anaphylaxis should always be considered when hypotension is temporarily related to the administration of a parenteral drug (Vitkun, 1997). Rapid recognition is essential because morbidity may be as high as 3% to 4% (Chung & Lam, 1997).

Anaphylaxis results from an antigen-antibody reaction that develops as a result of previous exposure to the antigen, such as a drug or protein, causing sensitization. Cross-sensitization may occur from a different substance that has a structure similar to that of the antigen (Chung & Lam, 1997). Conversely, there is no antibody involvement in an anaphylactoid reaction. Both types of reactions may occur within minutes of exposure, with severity ranging from mild urticaria to shock and death.

Histamine is released by mast cells in both types; however, the antigen-antibody reactions also cause release of leukotrienes, prostaglandins, and kinins. The following symptoms may manifest in the anesthetized patient suffering from an anaphylactic or anaphylactoid reaction.

- Urticaria
- Facial, oropharyngeal, or laryngeal edema
- Flushing
- Wheezing
- Bronchospasm
- Tachycardia
- Profound hypotension due to systemic vasodilation
- Cardiorespiratory collapse

Treatment, which must be rapid and comprehensive, includes these actions:

- Discontinue administration of the suspected cause if it can be identified quickly.
- Change to a different class of anesthetic agents if the cause of allergic reaction is unknown.
- Administer oxygen by face mask if there is no edema or airway obstruction, or intubate and control ventilation.
- Expand circulatory volume with IV fluids, bearing in mind that plasma volume expanders may be causative agents.
- Provide pharmacologic support, including:
  - IV epinephrine
  - IV aminophylline
  - IV diphenhydramine or cimetidine
  - IV corticosteroids.
- Conclude surgery as quickly as possible.

Epinephrine is very effective in treating anaphylaxis because of its ability to bind with alpha- and beta-adrenergic receptors, producing vasoconstriction, which increases blood pressure and heart rate. It also directly dilates the bronchi (Noble, 2005). Diphenhydramine, an H_1 histamine antagonist, and the H_2 histamine antagonists cimetidine and ranitidine do not inhibit the release of histamine by mast cells or basophils and cannot reverse an ongoing anaphylactic or anaphylactoid reaction (Chung & Lam, 1997). However, these antihistamines are able to block the effects of already released histamine at receptor sites. Corticosteroids stabilize mast cells, reducing the inflammatory reaction. Additionally, hydrocortisone has an added mineral corticoid effect that causes the reabsorption of sodium ions and water resulting in expansion of the blood volume (Noble, 2005).

Many agents commonly used in health care settings have been linked to anaphylactic and anaphylactoid reactions. Contrast media used in radiology is frequently associated with allergic reactions. Substances used during surgery, such as bone cement, dextrans, antibiotics, protamine, streptokinase, and blood products, may also cause allergic reactions. Anesthetic agents and ancillary drugs

Antaphylactic rxn - occurs only after the pt has been previously exposed at least once to the antigen + is sensitized. An Anaphylactoid rxn can occur after a single, first time exposure to certain agents in non sensitized patients. Both produce the same clinical manifestations + are treated the same.

may promote histamine release from mast cells in a nonimmunologic, dose-dependent manner (Vitkun, 1997). The following drugs may act as foreign substances that precipitate reactions.

- IV anesthetics – barbiturates, propofol, etomidate
- Muscle relaxants – especially the nondepolarizing type
- Opioids – morphine, meperidine, codeine, fentanyl
- Local anesthetics – those of the aminoester type, such as procaine

A thorough preoperative assessment is a key factor in identifying the patient who may be at risk so that preventive measures may be considered in perioperative planning. A known history of atopy, such as bronchial asthma, will be a consideration in the rapid differential diagnosis of the cause that must be made during surgery or anesthesia. Multiple surgical procedures (causing possible sensitization), reactions during dental or radiologic procedures, or episodes of related symptoms, including respiratory distress, are all important considerations.

For individuals identified as being predisposed to allergic reaction, intradermal tests, basophil histamine-release tests, and radioallergosorbent testing (RAST) may be used for evaluation. The RAST results are not as accurate for a specific antigen as those achieved with an intradermal test using an extract of an allergen. However, the RAST evaluates the number of antibodies produced by the immune system, and elevated levels of certain antibodies may identify particular allergies (Cleveland Clinic, 2006). Pharmacologic preoperative prophylaxis with histamine-release antagonists and corticosteroids may decrease the severity of a reaction.

Latex Sensitivity

According to the U.S. Food and Drug Administration (FDA), allergic reactions to latex (natural rubber) have continued to rise since the first alert was issued in 1991. Theories about the reason include the increasing use of latex-containing articles in medical and consumer products, manufacturing techniques, and an increase of latex particles in the air resulting from environmental conditions.

Contact dermatitis is one of the most frequent signs of latex sensitivity, but it is possible that 12% of intraoperative anaphylactic reactions may be due to latex allergy. During surgery, reactions may be more severe due to the lack of normal tissue barriers and direct contact with blood, mucous membranes, and tissues (Vitkun, 1997). Anaphylactic response to latex may be confused with reactions to other substances during surgery and anesthesia because the onset of symptoms may be delayed for more than an hour after exposure (Morgan, Mikhail, & Murray, 2006). In patients who have had multiple operations, delayed allergic reaction to latex may occur 15 minutes or more after exposure, so it is possible for anaphylaxis to develop in the PACU (Cowling & Haas, 2001).

Latex sensitivity appears to develop with repeated exposures. Although the incidence among health care workers is greater than the general population, patients who undergo frequent procedures that put them in contact with latex-containing medical devices have the greatest incidence of latex allergic reaction. Children with spina bifida, meningocele, and urogenital abnormalities and adults with spinal cord injuries are believed to be sensitized by frequent urinary catheterization, digital disimpaction with a latex-gloved finger, and multiple surgeries that expose mucosal, serosal, parenteral, and peritoneal membranes to latex (Bernstein, 1996). Incidence of latex sensitivity among children with spina bifida is believed to be 30% to 70% (American Society of Anesthesiologists [ASA], 2005). Type I hypersensitiviy is an IgE-mediated true allergic reaction (ASA, 2005; Nobel, 2005).

Symptoms of a reaction in an anesthetized patient are similar to those listed in the previous section. Symptoms in an awake patient may be localized or generalized and include:

- hives, urticaria
- pruritus
- rhinitis or watery, itchy eyes
- edema of the eyelids
- faintness
- shortness of breath
- wheezing
- nausea or vomiting
- abdominal cramps
- diarrhea
- anaphylaxis.

Routes of exposure to latex include skin, mucous membrane, inhalation, parenteral injection, ingestion, or wound inoculation. Type IV sensitivity, allergic contact dermatitis, is not life-threatening and occurs immediately upon skin contact with latex. Another type of latex-associated dermatitis, irritant dermatitis, is more likely due to sensitivity to chemicals used in the manufacture of latex items. This type of reaction takes from 6 to 72 hours to develop and produces irritated, dry, cracking skin (ASA, 2005).

Latex is used extensively in medical, surgical, and anesthetic equipment and devices. A few examples are gloves, tourniquets, syringes, IV fluid containers and delivery systems, catheters, endotracheal tubes, ventilator bellows, IV injection ports, face masks, blood pressure cuffs, and ID bracelets. A master list of latex-containing materials should be available in every ambulatory facility, as well as a list of safe alternatives. The FDA now requires latex content labeling of medical equipment, and some glove manufacturers must quantify the protein levels in the latex. Still, some of the latex protein leaches into the powder used with the gloves and when that powder gets into the air, it may remain airborne for 8 to 12 hours (ASA, 2005; Noble, 2005), ultimately settling on surfaces of equipment, drapes, gowns, and various items in the area.

When a patient is known or suspected to be sensitive to latex, stringent precautions must be taken and a latex-safe environment must be instituted. Precautions range from substituting drug ampules for vials with rubber stoppers (or removing rubber stoppers from vials) to covering equipment that cannot be substituted, such as monitors and wires, with stockinette taped in place. Ideally, the patient is scheduled as the first case, before latex dust accumulates in the air. Similar precautions must be taken in preoperative preparation and postoperative care. Each ambulatory surgical facility should have established policies and protocols for care of the latex-sensitive patient.

A thorough preoperative history, including possible occupational exposure and suggestive symptoms of latex allergy, is important so that precautions and preparations for a safe surgical procedure may be planned. The FDA recommends that patients be questioned about itching, rash, or wheezing after blowing up balloons or wearing latex gloves. However, a 1997 study of nearly 1,000 ambulatory surgical patients suggested that, although the 6.7% incidence of latex sensitivity found was a significant potential problem, history alone did not appear to be a reliable predictor of the presence of antilatex antibodies when compared with IgE serum levels as measured by the sensitive AlaSTAT test. The study also found that risk of latex allergy increased with male gender, non-Caucasian race, asthma, spinal cord abnormalities, certain food allergies, stated latex allergy, and symptom development when exposed to latex (Lebenbom-Mansour et al., 1997).

The efficacy of preoperative medication for prophylaxis of latex reaction has not been established, although H_1 and H_2 histamine antagonists and steroids may be beneficial. Patients need to be informed of suspected latex sensitivity and advised to make this known before future dental, surgical, or emergency procedures. Wearing a Medic-Alert indicator is advisable with documented latex sensitivity (Cleveland Clinic, 2006).

SUMMARY

The perianesthesia nurse's awareness and understanding of the variety and scope of serious and life-threatening complications that may occur at any time perioperatively is the best preventive measure for patient safety. Early recognition of impending complications followed by effective treatment is key to favorable patient outcomes.

EXAM QUESTIONS

CHAPTER 6

Questions 72-90

Note: Choose the option that BEST answers each question.

72. To facilitate abdominal laparoscopic surgery, the person performing the procedure intentionally creates a

    a. pneumothorax.
    b. pneumoperitoneum.
    c. crepitus.
    d. pneumonitis.

73. During laparoscopic surgery, the patient develops tachycardia, hypotension, cyanosis, and dysrhythmia. A likely cause is

    a. aspiration.
    b. hypervolemia.
    c. malignant hyperthermia (MH).
    d. gas embolus.

74. Routine analysis of the patient's expired carbon dioxide concentration during laparoscopic surgery may detect

    a. hypoxemia.
    b. aspiration.
    c. gas embolus.
    d. hyperkalemia.

75. If a gas embolus is suspected, the patient should immediately be given

    a. dantrolene.
    b. morphine.
    c. 100% oxygen.
    d. nitrous oxide.

76. Sudden bradycardia that develops during eye surgery is most likely due to

    a. eyelash reflex.
    b. celiac plexus reflex.
    c. oculocardiac reflex.
    d. sympathomimetic reflex.

77. Continuous monitoring of the heart rate during ophthalmic surgery is essential because of the danger of sudden

    a. tachycardia.
    b. bigeminy.
    c. bradycardia.
    d. celiac reflex.

78. Patients who have undergone nose, throat, or oral surgery are especially prone to

    a. nausea and vomiting.
    b. airway compromise.
    c. hypotension.
    d. hypovolemia.

79. Suction lipoplasty may be associated with

    a. significant blood loss.
    b. major fluid compartment shifts.
    c. systemic fluid absorption.
    d. gas embolus.

80. The Trendelenburg position may
    a. compromise ventilation.
    b. promote aspiration.
    c. increase nausea and vomiting.
    d. decrease venous return.

81. A possible complication following the use of a tourniquet is
    a. hemorrhage.
    b. hypertension.
    c. hypersensitivity.
    d. neurovascular injury.

82. Inhalation of foreign liquid or solid material into the tracheobronchial tree is
    a. asphyxiation.
    b. aspiration.
    c. respiration.
    d. regurgitation.

83. The systemic absorption of irrigating solutions during endoscopic procedures may cause
    a. electrolyte imbalance.
    b. pneumoperitoneum.
    c. diuresis.
    d. hemorrhage.

84. Aspirated solid material that obstructs areas of the tracheobronchial tree causes
    a. pneumonitis.
    b. crepitation.
    c. pneumothorax.
    d. atelectasis.

85. Patients with increased intra-abdominal pressure, such as obesity or pregnancy, have an increased perioperative risk of
    a. hypoxemia.
    b. aspiration.
    c. gas emboli.
    d. hyperkalemia.

86. An emergency method for delivering oxygen directly into the trachea is
    a. tracheoscopy.
    b. cricothyrotomy.
    c. bronchoscopy.
    d. laryngectomy.

87. Malignant hyperthermia (MH) occurs most commonly in
    a. older children and young adults.
    b. young children and elderly adults.
    c. children with spina bifida.
    d. women of childbearing age.

88. A drug specifically indicated for the treatment of malignant hyperthermia (MH) is
    a. metoclopramide (Reglan).
    b. flumazenil (Romazicon).
    c. sodium citrate (Bicitra).
    d. dantrolene (Dantrium).

89. Which substance is released in anaphylactic and anaphylactoid reactions?
    a. Leukotrienes
    b. Histamine
    c. Prostaglandins
    d. Kinins

90. Children with spina bifida exhibit a greater than normal incidence of

    a. nausea and vomiting.
    b. aspiration pneumonitis.
    c. postintubation croup.
    d. latex sensitivity.

CHAPTER 7

PEDIATRIC AND GERIATRIC CONSIDERATIONS

CHAPTER OBJECTIVE

Upon completion of this chapter, the reader will be able to identify unique considerations relative to pediatric and geriatric populations in the ambulatory surgical setting.

LEARNING OBJECTIVES

After studying this chapter, the reader will be able to:

1. identify the emotional needs of pediatric patients at various ages.
2. select appropriate perioperative nursing interventions for pediatric ambulatory surgery patients.
3. identify nursing interventions that enhance the well-being and safety of geriatric patients perioperatively.
4. discuss postoperative cognitive dysfunction in older patients.

INTRODUCTION

One of the challenges of ambulatory surgical nursing is the need to care for a variety of patients with special needs who, if hospitalized, would be cared for by specialists. Age-specific and disease-associated recommendations and precautions are offered throughout this course, but there are special considerations for pediatric and geriatric patients that the perioperative nurse should understand and consider in order to provide a safe and pleasant ambulatory surgical experience. Some of these considerations are presented in this chapter.

PEDIATRIC PATIENTS

The number of pediatric surgical procedures performed in ambulatory settings continues to grow, due in part to the patient benefits. As outpatients, children are spared the anxiety and fears associated with being separated from their families, and have minimal disruption of their comfortable daily routine. Because of the large number of pediatric ambulatory procedures done, some ambulatory facilities are devoted exclusively to children and are staffed by professionals specializing in pediatrics.

However, most ambulatory surgical facilities treat adult and pediatric patients. Because the physiologic, anatomic, and pharmacologic characteristics of neonates, infants, and young children are considerably different than those of adolescents and young adults, the perioperative nurse should be familiar with normal ranges and values for vital signs and other parameters to develop an appropriate care plan and recognize deviations that may require intervention.

For example, determining the pediatric patient's weight in kilograms (divide pounds by 2.2) is an important safety precaution considering medication dosages and intravenous (IV) fluid requirements are calculated in kilograms. Kilogram scales are available that eliminate the possibility of conversion errors. Dosages should be carefully checked before administration, and any order that seems inappropriate should be questioned.

Psychological Preparation

A patient's psychological needs vary with his or her age; as children grow older, their concerns and reactions to the prospect of surgery change.

The first 3 years are the most vulnerable. Too young to understand what will be done, they are old enough to remember the procedure. An unpleasant surgical experience may cause subsequent visits to the doctor or hospital setting to be stressful challenges for the child and parents.

Separation anxiety is greatest in this age-group. Parents should be cautioned not to say good-bye, but rather to tell the child they will be waiting in another room. Children, especially up to 4 years of age, need frequent reassurance that parents are waiting. This age-group benefits from examining (handling) strange new equipment and the use of "magical" equipment. They should also be allowed to bring a favorite toy or stuffed animal with them to the facility.

From 4 to 7 years, separation anxiety is less intense for children because they are better able to understand that parents will be waiting. However, they also understand that something is going to be done to their body, which is a frightening thought.

Throughout the preoperative phase, parent's attitudes strongly influence the child's reaction and behavior. Children take their cues from their parents, so an anxious parent may result in an anxious child. Parents should talk openly and in a matter-of-fact manner about what is going to happen. When the child discerns that the surgery is nothing to fear because the parents are not upset, the preparation is more likely to be better accepted and less stressful.

Children in the 4- to 7-year age-group benefit from rehearsing and role-playing, but they are still young enough to be comforted by a favorite toy. They are curious about new things (e.g., equipment) and will either believe or laugh at the idea of magical effects.

During the school years, children are learning and developing their self-esteem. Surgery may be interpreted as a threat to the integrity of their bodies, so they may need to feel they have some control over circumstances associated with the surgical experience. A preoperative visit to the ambulatory surgery facility is especially helpful to this age-group. It gives them a chance to ask questions (control) and investigate.

Adolescents tend to give the impression that they do not care, yet they are very concerned about the details of the surgery, especially if it will affect their body image. Independence is important to them; they may prefer not to have a parent assist them. They value privacy and confidentiality and are more prone to honestly answer personal questions, such as drug use, if parents are not present.

Regardless of the patient's age, parents assume considerable responsibility for pediatric ambulatory surgical patients and may be quietly overwhelmed. They must be integrated into the care plan and well informed. Many facilities provide age-appropriate books and video tapes that can be used in the home setting to teach patients and parents as they prepare for surgery.

One of the most difficult things for a parent is to relinquish care to the perioperative staff. Parents should be made to feel that their trust is well placed and that the child's well-being and safety are the staff's primary concern. They must be well informed about perioperative proceedings and understand that complying with preoperative and postoperative instructions is essential to a safe and uneventful surgery.

Immediate Preoperative Preparation

Preoperative Food and Fluid Intake

Children should be scheduled as early in the day as possible to avoid the irritability and dehydration associated with withholding food and liquids. The trend is to liberalize oral restrictions. This process may mean no intake of solids or milk products permitted 6 to 8 hours before surgery, but clear liquids would be allowed until 3 hours before surgery for children ages 7 months to through adolescence (Cote, 2002).

To avoid dehydration, infants and toddlers may be encouraged to take clear liquids 2 to 3 hours before the scheduled surgery, even if they must be awakened to do so. Breast milk is not considered a clear fluid; it contains considerable fat that activates the digestive process, causing increased gastric acid (Yemen, 1998). The 3-hour clear fluid restriction allows for last-minute schedule changes, permitting patients to be moved up as long as they have been on nothing-by-mouth (NPO) status for clear fluids for at least 2 hours (Cote, 2002). Increasingly, for short procedures under local anesthesia NPO is not mandated.

Premedication

It is generally agreed that the best premedication for a pediatric patient is a calm, supportive parent. For this reason, allowing a parent to be with the child during anesthetic induction may permit omission or reduction of sedative or anxiolytic premedication. Omitting premedication for pediatric outpatients usually results in a more speedy return to preoperative status or home readiness.

Parent participation is at the discretion of the anesthesia provider and the policy of the facility (Cote, 2005). The child's expected response during anesthetic induction must be explained to the parent in great detail, so that the parent may decide if he or she will be able to accept the experience without interference. Although parents often request participation, most are unaware of the child's response to induction under inhalation anesthesia and many individuals are not able to remain calm as they watch, which may be disruptive rather than beneficial.

Available as a syrup, oral midazolam is the most commonly used pediatric premedication in the United States (Cote, 2005). Other liquid oral medications given with a small amount of sweet liquid, are usually well tolerated. For inconsolable or combative children, intramuscular (IM) ketamine may be chosen to facilitate separation from the parents and transition into anesthetic induction. Nose drops are another option that may be used with drugs such as midazolam, ketamine, or sufentanil.

An alternative route for small children weighing less than 20 kg is rectal administration. Methohexital (Brevital) is usually effective within 10 minutes. Midazolam may also be given rectally, but it may prolong recovery. Regardless of which sedative is administered, the child should never be left unattended. Airway obstruction, coughing, and hiccups may develop. In addition to the possibility of oversedation, a disadvantage associated with rectal administration is defecation and expulsion of an unknown amount of drug before it is absorbed. Taping the buttocks together may help to prevent expulsion.

Anticholinergic medications, such as atropine, scopolamine, or glycopyrrolate (Robinul) are commonly given preoperatively to decrease the possibility of bradycardia occurring during some surgical procedures or general anesthesia induction. These drugs also reduce respiratory secretions. Transdermal scopolamine is believed to be beneficial in preventing nausea and vomiting, especially if related to motion, and may be prescribed for ambulatory patients. Although perioperative staff should be monitoring premedicated patients, parents who may also be with the child should be cautioned not to let a premedicated child run and jump.

Intraoperative Phase

Before any pediatric procedure is started, appropriately sized equipment must be available, including monitoring devices and emergency equipment. Adult-size blood pressure cuffs, pulse oximetry sensors, and even stethoscopes will not provide accurate information. Most importantly, an assortment of pediatric-size airways, masks, and other ventilatory support equipment must be at the site of all preoperative, intraoperative, and postoperative care.

Toddlers are commonly anesthetized to the point of unconsciousness while sitting on the anesthesia provider's lap. Young children may be given the option of sitting or lying on the operating table. They are typically allowed to hold the mask themselves; volatile inhalation anesthetics produce unconsciousness within minutes. Older children may accept venipuncture for IV induction. EMLA cream, an eutetic mixture of local anesthetics, applied to the skin may make the venipuncture more acceptable. However, it must be applied 1 hour before venipuncture to be effective. Lidocaine iontophoresis, which uses electrical stimulation, reduces the onset time to 10 minutes and increases the depth of dermal anesthesia to 6.4 mm in that time versus 5 mm maximum with EMLA. Some children may occasionally find itching, tingling, or burning sensations distressing (Pasero, 2006). Supplemental regional anesthesia decreases the general anesthetic requirement and provides preemptive pain control for the postoperative period.

Postoperative Phase

Pediatric patients require diligent postoperative monitoring. Respiratory complications are more common in children than in adults, so unless contraindicated by the surgery, children should be placed on their sides to allow secretions or blood to drain from the mouth as a precaution against aspiration or laryngospasm. As reflexes return, laryngospasm may be caused by secretions irritating the vocal cords. For surgical procedures that require tracheal intubation, the child should be extubated either before the cough reflex returns or after protective reflexes have returned, which is usually when the child is alert enough to open his or her eyes.

Postoperative nausea and vomiting (PONV) is frequently more problematic in pediatric patients, largely due to the types of surgery performed in ambulatory settings, such as strabismus correction and orchiopexy, and inhalation anesthesia. The trend toward not requiring fluid intake until the child asks for something to drink helps to reduce the incidence, but medication may be required if nausea or vomiting is severe or protracted. Children are more prone to agitation and other parkinsonian side effects associated with antiemetics, and they should be carefully observed for these before discharge (Yemen, 1998). For children who have had throat surgery, such as a tonsillectomy, analgesic rectal suppositories are an effective option to oral medication considering the surgery associated swallowing and possible PONV.

The amount of pain experienced by different children who have undergone similar surgical procedures differs widely. Children have fluctuating analgesia requirements, so an effective pain management plan should include provisions for breakthrough pain (Brislin & Rose, 2005).

Pain management in children may be compromised by the difficulty in assessing its severity, especially in the very young. Depending on age, behavior assessment, distraction techniques, or visual picture scales may be effective. For nonverbal children or those with cognitive impairment, the caregiver should be assisted in developing an individualized numeric rating scale for their child's pain behaviors. As shown in Figure 7-1, this assessment can be done using facial expressions, leg activity, arm activity, crying, and consolability (FLACC) and is usable through out recovery and convalescence (Brislin & Rose, 2005). Again, in the Phase II setting, the presence of a parent may reduce both physiologic and psychologic distress.

Children old enough to understand should be told before surgery that they will awaken in a dif-

FIGURE 7-1: FLACC BEHAVIORAL PAIN SCALE

Categories	Scoring 0	1	2
Face	No particular expression or smile	Occasional grimace or frown, withdrawn, disinterested	Frequent to constant frown, clenched jaw, quivering chin
Legs	Normal position or relaxed	Uneasy, restless, tense	Kicking, or legs drawn up
Activity	Lying quietly, normal position, moves easily	Squirming, shifting back and forth, tense	Arched, rigid, or jerking
Cry	No cry (awake or asleep)	Moans or whimpers, occasional complaint	Crying steadily, screams or sobs, frequent complaints
Consolability	Content, relaxed	Reassured by occasional touching, hugging, or being talked to, distractable	Difficult to console or comfort

Each of the five categories (F) Face; (L) Legs; (A) Activity; (C) Cry; (C) Consolability is scored from 0-2, which results in a total score between zero and ten.

Pain Scale Instruction:

Patients who are awake: Observe for at least 2-5 minutes. Observe legs and body uncovered. Reposition patient or observe activity, assess body for tenseness and tone. Initiate consoling interventions if needed

Patients who are asleep: Observe for at least 5 minutes or longer. Observe body and legs uncovered. If possible reposition the patient. Touch the body and assess for tenseness and tone.

Face
- Score 0 point if patient has a relaxed face, eye contact and interest in surroundings
- Score 1 point if patient has a worried look to face, with eyebrows lowered, eyes partially closed, cheeks raised, mouth pursed
- Score 2 points if patient has deep furrows in the forehead, with closed eyes, open mouth and deep lines around nose/lips

Legs
- Score 0 points if patient has usual tone and motion to limbs (legs and arms)
- Score 1 point if patient has increase tone, rigidity, tense, intermittent flexion/extension of limbs
- Score 2 points if patient has hyper tonicity, legs pulled tight, exaggerated flexion/extension of limbs, tremors

Activity
- Score 0 points if patient moves easily and freely, normal activity/restrictions
- Score 1 point if patient shifts positions, hesitant to move, guarding, tense torso, pressure on body part
- Score 2 points if patient is in fixed position, rocking, side-to-side head movement, rubbing body part

Cry
- Score 0 points if patient has no cry/moan awake or asleep
- Score 1 point if patient has occasional moans, cries, whimpers, sighs
- Score 2 points if patient has frequent/continuous moans, cries, grunts

Consolability
- Score 0 points if patient is calm and does not require consoling
- Score 1 point if patient responds to comfort by touch or talk in ½- 1 minute
- Score 2 points if patient requires constant comforting or unable to console

Whenever feasible, behavioral measurement of pain should be used in conjunction with self-report. When self-report is not possible, interpretation of pain behaviors and decision making regarding treatment of pain requires careful consideration of the context in which the pain behaviors were observed.

Each category is scored on the 0-2 scale which results in a total score of 0-10

Assessment of Behavioral Score:

0 = Relaxed and comfortable
1-3 = Mild discomfort
4-6 = Moderate pain
7-10 = Severe discomfort/pain

Note. From Merkel, S., Voepel-Lewis, T., Shayevitz, J., & Malviya, S., 1997, The FLACC: A behavioral scale for scoring postoperative pain in young children. *Pediatric Nursing 1997, 23*:293-297. Reprinted with permission.

ferent room and see unfamiliar faces. Nevertheless, this is a frightening experience. Some facilities allow one parent to be with the child in Phase II and step-down areas, which benefits the child and parent. Disorientation, hallucinations, and uncontrollable movements may occur during emergence from general anesthesia, possibly due to pain, sensory deprivation, or the unknown environment. In some cases, irritability and hyperactivity may last up to 24 hours (Lancaster, 1997).

Discharge

Parents are often anxious about their ability to provide adequate care postoperatively. Detailed written and verbal instructions, including what to observe for and what actions to take, plus telephone numbers for questions and emergencies should be provided. Ideally, comprehensive written instructions in nonmedical language should be given to parents on a preoperative visit to the doctor or the ambulatory facility. Although these instructions should be explained again on the day of surgery before discharge, parents are stressed and anxious then, and have had to already make the appropriate arrangements. Parents should have received postoperative prescriptions prior to the day of surgery so they do not have to stop at a pharmacy on the way home from the facility. They should be alerted that fever within 24 hours of surgery and general anesthesia is a common problem (Lancaster, 1997). One of the advantages of ambulatory surgery for pediatric patients is that postoperative circumstances allow patients to be active, which encourages deep breathing and may help reduce fever.

Because motion of the automobile during the drive home may provoke or exacerbate nausea and vomiting, parents should be prepared. For small children still marginally somnolent, it is important that parents be alerted that the child's airway may be dangerously compromised if the head slumps forward when the child is secured in a car seat. For all young children, a responsible adult should be seated next to the child to monitor head position to ensure airway patency and deal with possible secretions or vomitus during the trip home. As with all ambulatory surgical patients, parents should receive a follow-up phone call the next day.

Respiratory Complications

Postintubation Croup

An important cause of airway obstruction, postintubation croup may develop in young children as a result of edema of the glottis or trachea. Children between the ages of 1 to 4 years and those with Down syndrome are most prone to develop this complication. Postintubation croup is associated with repeated intubation attempts, size of the endotracheal tube used, duration of surgery, head and neck procedures, and excessive movement of the endotracheal tube as may occur with moving the patient's head or coughing while the tube is in place (Morgan, Mikhail, & Murphy, 2006). Treatment consists of aerosolized racemic epinephrine inhalation, a moist atmosphere, and possibly IV corticosteroid therapy.

Because the vasoconstriction produced by racemic epinephrine may dissipate within 2 hours, edema and obstruction may recur, even more severely. Consequently, it is essential to closely monitor the child during this period (Ireland, 2006). Ideally, children who have been intubated should be monitored in the postanesthesia care unit (PACU) for at least 3 hours, the period in which postintubation croup is most likely to occur.

Postobstructive Pulmonary Edema

Although relatively uncommon, the frequency of postobstructive pulmonary edema has been increasing over the past several years for unknown reasons. It has been associated with laryngospasm complicated by significant hypoxia in infants, but the exact cause is unknown. Treatment consists of supportive oxygen therapy, with continuous positive airway pressure and intubation if necessary (Yemen, 1998). The edema usually resolves over several hours, but overnight admission is advisable. Pulmonary edema has also been associated with nasal surgery, possibly due to vasoactive drugs (Yemen, 1998).

Pediatric Obstructive Sleep Apnea

As with adults in the United States, the number of overweight children has been steadily increasing. Overweight children are prone to airway problems. For example, approximately 20% of obese children have obstructive sleep apnea (OSA), and as much as 3% of all children have OSA. African American children have a 3% to 9% incidence. For pre-adolescents the incidence may be as high as 10% to 12% (Brown, K., 2005).

The intermittent episodes of hypoxemia and hypercarbia experienced during sleep adversely affect the quality of life and may have long-term effects for pediatric patients. Investigators have found that grade school children in the lowest tenth percentile have an OSA rate six to nine times greater than those in higher percentiles (Brown, K., 2005). Additionally, comorbidities of children with OSA may include asthma, chronic lower tract respiratory infections, systemic hypertension, pulmonary hypertension, and left ventricular dysfunction. Symptoms of pediatric OSA include hyperactivity, poor concentration, snoring, enuresis, nocturnal mouth breathing, nightmares, earaches, and developmental delay (Olmas, 2007).

The American Academy of Pediatrics recommends that all children be screened for snoring and those at high-risk of OSA be referred to a sleep specialist and possibly to undergo a polysomnogram, considered the most accurate diagnostic tool. The Academy also recommends tonsillectomy and adenoidectomy (T&A), with re-evaluation after surgery (Bachenberg, 2005). Although a T&A may be curative for some cases of pediatric OSA, these children have a high incidence of complications postoperatively. Oxygen desaturation may occur as late as 8 hours after the procedure, which may be due to an inflammatory response that developed overtime due to snoring.

Children with OSA who have undergone coblation T&A had significantly better postoperative recovery. They required less pain medication and experienced fewer complications. However, regardless of surgical technique, all children younger than age 3 years are more prone to complications after tonsillectomy (Ellis, 2006).

Pediatric OSA patients require constant monitoring after surgery, and those with severe OSA, significant medical comorbidities, or upper respiratory infections are not suitable for ambulatory surgery (Brown, K., 2005).

GERIATRIC PATIENTS

By the year 2030, at least 20% of the United States population will be older than 65, and of these one of four individuals will be older than 85 years of age. Twenty-one percent of those older than 60 will have surgery and anesthesia versus only 12% of individuals in the 45 to 60 age-group (Liu & Leung, 2006). Just as children should not be considered miniature adults, older adults should not be considered feeble adults. Although some geriatric patients may be fragile and need gentle care, they deserve respect and emotional support. Some may also need a nursing advocate. Preoperative teaching is particularly important to allay fears and improve postoperative cooperation. Learning may take longer in older patients and sensory impairments and environmental distraction should be considered during teaching (McEwen, 2003).

Older patients benefit from avoiding hospitalization in many ways: less opportunity for becoming disoriented due to unfamiliar surroundings, decreased exposure to infection, decreased likelihood of serious postoperative respiratory complications caused by inactivity, and less upset of comfortable daily routines.

Although a generalized decline in systemic function inevitably occurs with advancing age, physiologic age (functional status) is more predictive than chronologic age. The healthy, alert, active individual is more likely to tolerate the stresses associated with surgery and anesthesia than is the stereotypical infirm individual, regardless of chronological age. Age-related disease, not age itself, is primarily responsible for morbidity and mortality in older patients (Liu & Leung, 2006; McLeskey, 2006). For example, atherosclerosis is pathologic; it is not found in healthy older patients (Morgan, Mikhail, & Murphy, 2006). Factors that increase surgical risk are related to systemic disease, functional abilities, mental health, and nutritional status.

Nevertheless, the normal aging process causes a decreased margin of reserve in organ function, resulting in less adaptability. Loss of tissue elasticity alters cardiovascular hemodynamics and pulmonary function. Decrease in lung elasticity allows overdistention of the alveoli and collapse of small airways resulting in decreased efficiency of air exchange. The effect of these emphysema-like changes may decrease arterial oxygenation on average 0.35 mm Hg per year (Morgan, Mikhail, & Murray, 2006). Reduced arterial compliance results in increased afterload, elevated systolic blood pressure, and left ventricular hypertrophy. Although cardiac output typically declines with age, it may be maintained in well-conditioned healthy individuals (Morgan, Mikhail, & Murphy, 2006).

Coronary artery disease is frequently found in older patients. In men, the incidence increases in a linear fashion from 50 to 80 years of age, whereas in women it is most likely to be seen after menopause. In a study of perioperative ischemia, coronary artery disease was found to be a predictive factor of postoperative myocardial ischemia, which is associated with adverse events such as myocardial infarction and death. Other predictors include left ventricular hypertrophy, hypertension, diabetes mellitus, and digoxin therapy. Incidence of postoperative myocardial ischemia ranged from 22% in patients with none of these predictors to 97% in patients with four of the five factors (Krechel, 1997).

Hepatic and renal blood flow and tissue mass decrease result in slower biotransformation of drugs and delayed elimination. Eventually, functional reserve declines more rapidly after the age of 80. Many geriatric surgical patients have mild to severe metabolic and hemodynamic deficits.

Aging increases perception thresholds, including vision, hearing, touch, smell, temperature, and proprioception. Still, pain is extensively processed; it may be inappropriate to routinely withhold treatment for pain and anxiety to avoid drug-induced complications. Alteration in subtypes of pain perception does not mean there is a decreased need for analgesia (Cook & Rooke, 2003). Unrelenting pain, rather than analgesics, may be responsible for postoperative delirium and agitation (Krechel, 1997). However, because of cerebral synaptic changes that affect short-term memory, even minimal perioperative sedation may cause amnesia or disorientation for extended periods of time, which may be problematic for outpatients (Muravchick, 1997).

Postoperative confusion and mental dysfunction are major concerns in older patients. Surgery as an outpatient may reduce the incidence and severity of these occurrences because the patients will be given fewer medications and be able to return to their normal surroundings within hours. The lack of control a hospitalized patient has adversely affects the emotional state, performance, subjective well-being, and physiologic function in older patients. An outpatient setting with less loss of control and autonomy should be beneficial (McLeskey, 2006).

Cognitive dysfunction is a deterioration of psychomotor abilities such as memory, central processing time, and acquisition of new information that is common in geriatric patients after surgery

(Cook & Rooke, 2003). Postoperative cognitive deficit (POCD) varies widely, but is associated with increasing age, duration of the procedure and anesthesia, lack of education, repeat surgery, postoperative infections, and respiratory infections (Barnett, 2001; Liu & Leung, 2006).

However, a history of neurologic disease or chronic factors, such as vision or hearing loss, depression, subclinical dementia, and alcoholism, increases risk. POCD is considered a mild neurocognitive disorder, and the diagnosis can only be established if the cognitive decline can be substantiated by the results of neuropsychological testing; preferably preoperatively and postoperatively. The testing must show that the patient has new onset of cognitive deficits in a minimum of two areas of cognitive function that lasts for 2 weeks or longer after surgery (Monk, 2004).

Delirium is a fluctuating level of consciousness that may occur postoperatively and may last for more than a week. However, this condition is more associated with other medical complications, prolonged hospitalization, or decreased functional status on discharge (Cook & Rooke, 2003). Cerebral ischemia is a major cause of delirium during recovery that may result from hypotension, hyperventilation, or hypoxia. Primary vascular causes include transient ischemic attacks or strokes. However, if the delirium does not respond to oxygen therapy or the correction of other possible clinical causes, then treatment may be as simple as returning eyeglasses or restoring a hearing aid to the patient, or allowing family members into the PACU (Krechel, 1997). Any or all of these factors play an important role in the patient's coping methods and adaptation to the everyday environment.

Postoperative delirium may occur with the use of regional or general anesthesia in the older patient (Muravchick, 2002). Because no particular anesthetic agent or technique has been definitively implicated, avoiding polypharmacy, an often unrecognized concern in geriatric patients, by minimizing the number of medications used, avoiding hypoxemia and hypercarbia, and providing adequate postoperative pain control appear to be the safest ways to minimize the possibility of postoperative mental dysfunction (Liu & Leung, 2006; Cook & Rooke, 2003).

In general, geriatric patients require lower doses of barbiturates, opioids, and benzodiazepines than other patients. With increasing age, there is a decrease in skeletal muscle mass, causing an increase in the proportion of total body fat. Consequently, fat-soluble drugs accumulate in tissues and the brain, resulting in delayed elimination. Due to this delay, diazepam may cause confusion for days (Morgan, Mikhail, & Murphy, 2006). Older patients have a comparable level of sedation with diazepam at plasma levels significantly lower than in younger patients (McLeskey, 2006).

Geriatric patients, particularly if malnourished, may also have decreased plasma proteins. With less protein available to bind to, more of the administered drug is unbound in the plasma, resulting in increased effect. Albumin, which tends to bind acidic drugs such as barbiturates and benzodiazepines, usually decreases with age, so the dosage of these drugs should be reduced for geriatric patients. For example, midazolam has been shown to be 94% protein bound so if there is a 20% reduction in albumin, the amount of drug free in the plasma is increased fourfold (Krechel, 1997). Similarly, meperidine is normally less protein bound than morphine, resulting in a more enhanced effect when plasma proteins are decreased. However, the biotransformations of drugs such as cistracurium, which has an organ-independent metabolism, are not affected by aging (Muravchick, 2002).

In addition, because of slower circulation time, the full effect of an IV medication may be delayed in older patients. To prevent overdosage, sufficient time should be allowed to observe and evaluate the effect of an IV medication before any additional administration.

Preoperative Preparation

A well-conducted preoperative assessment is essential for the aging patient. Mental status, general mood, and attitude toward surgery should be considered when planning perioperative care; the nursing history can reveal age-related changes and coexisting diseases (McEwen, 2003). Diminished thirst, poor nutrition, and diuretic medication may cause dehydration, which must be considered for intraoperative fluid management.

Older patients may be on several prescription medications and often neglect to mention over-the-counter medications, so these possibilities must be investigated and documented in the preoperative assessment. Another caution is that lidocaine iontophoresis should not be used to anesthetize venipuncture sites for patients with pacemakers or other electrically sensitive devices (Pasero, 2006).

Intraoperative Phase

The required concentration of the inhalation anesthetics halothane, isoflurane, and desflurane to produce anesthesia decreases linearly with age (McLeskey, 2006). The requirement for most inhalation anesthetics decreases by 30% from age 20 to age 80, and the average 80-year-old needs less than half the dose of thiopental for anesthetic induction than does a 20-year-old (Morgan, Mikhail, & Murphy, 2006). Similarly, the induction dose of barbiturates in a 70-year-old is approximately 30% less than that of a 20- to 30-year old (McLeskey, 2006).

Elderly patients have a 50% to 70% lower dose requirement for remifentanil due to decreased central clearance and distribution, which slows equilibration (Egan, 2001). Propofol also requires a significant dose reduction; older patients are 30% to 50% more sensitive to propofol than are younger adults (Cook & Rooke, 2003). Consequently, for patients with deteriorating mental status, the use of multiple medications may compromise prompt recovery to the preoperative level, which is particularly important for the older ambulatory surgery patient.

Unless regional anesthesia is supplemented with moderate to heavy sedation, postoperative confusion may be less than after general anesthesia. With spinal anesthesia, postdural puncture headache is less likely to occur, but urinary retention is more likely. Regardless of the anesthetic technique used, any sudden or prolonged drop in blood pressure may lead to hypoxemia, myocardial or cerebral ischemia, infarction, thrombosis, or embolism (Burns, 1996). However, cerebrovascular accident is a rare perioperative complication despite the wide fluctuations in blood pressure that may occur during anesthesia and surgery (Muravchick, 1997).

Intraoperative hypothermia may cause postoperative vasoconstriction and shivering, resulting in increased oxygen consumption that may predispose the patient to myocardial ischemia. During anesthesia, the core body rate of an elderly patient decreases more than twice as fast as that of a young adult (Muravchick, 1997). Fragile skin and limited joint mobility require special care to avoid trauma from improper positioning. Decreased immune responsiveness is also associated with aging, which increases susceptibility to infection and sepsis.

Postoperative Phase

For patients of advanced age, general and spinal anesthesia are associated with decreased body temperature. The higher the level of anesthesia achieved with spinal anesthesia, the greater the decrease in core temperature. Unintentional hypothermia has been related to myocardial ischemia, angina, and hypoxemia, especially in high-risk patients having lower extremity vascular surgery (Sieber & Pauldine, 2005). Hypothermia is known to increase the stress response to surgery and may interfere with coagulation (Pasero, 2006).

In the PACU, older patients require careful monitoring due to their diminished ventilatory responses to hypoxia or hypercarbia. Aging produces a twofold increase in the risk of airway obstruction, hypoxemia, or carbon dioxide retention (Muravchick, 1997). Older patients are more prone to cardiovascular and central nervous system events perioperatively, but have less nausea, shivering, and dizziness than younger adults (Barnett, 2001). Postoperatively, ventilatory problems are disproportionately more common in elderly patients (Cook & Rooke, 2003). Aspiration pneumonia is a common and potentially life-threatening complication in the elderly, largely due to decreased protective laryngeal reflexes (Morgan, Mikhail, & Murphy, 2006). Patients suffering from Parkinson's disease have additional problems due to difficulty in swallowing and managing secretions along with often-decreased respiratory effort.

Many older patients live with chronic lung disease, so a primary concern during the immediate and extended postoperative period is to facilitate adequate respiration and prevent dyspnea.

To prevent atelectasis, it is essential that older patients be able to cough to keep the airway clear. Ineffective coughing consumes energy and oxygen and may lead to dyspnea. Instructing patients in controlled cough after several deep breaths, while supporting the operative site if appropriate, should prove helpful. Perhaps more easily remembered by the patient is "huff" coughing. In this method, after a deep breath the patient audibly "huffs" on expiration (Geiger-Bronsky, 1998). However, this method requires the use of abdominal muscles during expiration and may be too uncomfortable immediately postoperatively for certain procedures, even with support of the incision.

Self-care management strategies need to be emphasized in the PACU before discharge. Pursed-lip breathing is an easily taught method that has been shown to be effective in minimizing dyspnea and maintaining adequate oxygen saturation in patients with chronic obstructive and restrictive lung disease (Geiger-Bronsky, 1998). Simple, deliberate deep sighing may be helpful in promoting lung expansion.

Discharge

For many older patients who live alone, the postdischarge recovery period may require assistance from community health care sources. Similarly, for couples, the person who undergoes ambulatory surgery may be the primary caregiver in the relationship and will have no reliable adult support after discharge. Both of these circumstances require the nurse to act as advocate for the patient and ensure that adequate care will be provided when the patient leaves the ambulatory facility. The challenge for nurses is to identify, plan, and provide nursing care to meet the needs of each patient (McEwen, 2003). To create a safe discharge plan, the nurse must find a balance between the patient's normal circumstances and the resources that are available and acceptable to the individual (Burden, 2004).

A responsible adult who will remain with the patient overnight must accompany the patient home and preferably remain with the patient to monitor the extended recovery period (Morgan, Mikhail, & Murray, 2006). These arrangements should have been finalized preoperatively. Written and verbal instructions should be provided. Large print instructions may be helpful for older patients. It is important that the responsible caregiver, as well as the patient, verbally demonstrate an understanding of these instructions because residual effects of medications may affect the patient's recall.

In addition, the patient and responsible adult should be provided with a 24-hour emergency phone number and cautioned about the signs to monitor for and the actions to take should they occur. The patient should receive a follow-up phone call the next morning. With adequate planning and preparation, the older patient should benefit from the minimal upset of daily routine that ambulatory surgery provides.

SUMMARY

The most fragile patients are found in the pediatric and geriatric age-groups, the extremes of the patient population. Ambulatory procedures offer significant benefits for both age-groups, but each requires special nursing skills and a patient-care focused environment for an optimal outcome.

EXAM QUESTIONS

CHAPTER 7

Questions 91-96

Note: Choose the option that BEST answers each question.

91. A medication administered preoperatively to decrease oral and respiratory secretions is

    a. metoclopramide.
    b. midazolam.
    c. atropine.
    d. morphine.

92. To decrease the possibility of bradycardia during general anesthesia induction and certain surgical procedures, a child may be given which drug preoperatively?

    a. Meprobamate
    b. Midazolam
    c. Atropine
    d. Morphine

93. For young children, general anesthesia is usually induced by

    a. intravenous injection.
    b. inhalation.
    c. rectal suppository.
    d. topical application.

94. Because of the possibility of developing postintubation croup, children who have been intubated should be monitored in the postanesthesia care unit for a minimum of

    a. 1 hour.
    b. 2 hours.
    c. 3 hours.
    d. 4 hours.

95. In older patients, postoperative cognitive dysfunction may be minimized by avoiding postoperative

    a. hypertension.
    b. hyperkalemia.
    c. polypharmacy.
    d. nausea and vomiting.

96. During the postoperative period, geriatric patients are especially vulnerable to

    a. anaphylaxis.
    b. hyperglycemia.
    c. ventilatory problems.
    d. hyperthermia.

CHAPTER 8

RISK MANAGEMENT, PATIENT SAFETY, AND QUALITY IMPROVEMENT

CHAPTER OBJECTIVE

Upon completion of this chapter, the reader will be able to explain how patient safety, risk management, and quality improvement are integral parts of perioperative practice.

LEARNING OBJECTIVES

After studying this chapter, the reader will be able to

1. identify outcomes to be expected from a risk management program.
2. explain the differences between risk management and quality improvement.
3. discuss the need for meticulous documentation
4. discuss the nurse's role in quality improvement.

INTRODUCTION

The expanding scope of nursing in the health care system brings with it added responsibilities. Contemporary nurses are expected to assess, plan for, recognize, and interpret clinical occurrences and determine appropriate interventions. Consequently, awareness of patient safety, risk management, and quality improvement issues, along with involvement in these processes, is essential for the perioperative nurse. An in-depth discussion of these issues is beyond the scope of this chapter. The information presented is intended as an introduction to raise awareness.

RISK MANAGEMENT

The primary goals of any ambulatory procedure are patient safety and satisfaction. Preventing or reducing patient and staff injury may be expected to reduce the liability and financial loss associated with malpractice litigation. Risk management and quality improvement are closely related but not synonymous. Preventing incidents or injuries is the focus of risk management, whereas quality improvement focuses on provision of health care and patterns of practice. Risk management is involved with standards of care that at least meet minimum legal requirements, whereas quality assurance may enhance standards. Both practices result in improved patient care.

Risk Identification, Analysis, and Control

As with the Surgical Care Improvement Project, a national quality improvement initiative whose goal is to use evidence-based actions to reduce preventable surgical complications by 25% by 2010 (American College of Surgeons, 2006), application of a risk management program on a departmental/facility basis requires development and implementation of mechanisms aimed at risk identification, analysis, and control (Kost, 2004). In the past, risk identification occurred when an incident was reported; however, the concept of an incident is no longer only manifested as an injury, but it includes any event that might have resulted in injury. Analysis involves investigation and assessment to determine where and why the break in protocol occurred. Control involves taking the necessary actions to correct the breakdown. These actions should be consistent with state statutes, regulations of accrediting bodies, accepted standards of care, practices recommended by appropriate professional organizations, and recommended practice guidelines.

Well before any reporting of incidents or rescue of injured patients is required, the entire staff should be concerned about prevention. The ambulatory surgery setting has inherent dangers related to unconscious patients, dangerous medications and anesthetic agents, surgical interventions, and highly technical equipment, so prevention must be a key focus. Some specific areas of concern include ensuring proper patient identification, operative site identification, that all team members are attentive to the final "time out" prior to a procedure, medication safety, proper monitoring during and after sedation, and identification of patient allergies. The potential for fire and burns with the use of equipment and the need for adult support upon discharge must also be addressed.

Should a patient-related event occur, after appropriate action has been taken to administer any needed clinical care to the person or persons involved, any equipment or supplies that may have been involved (including disposable equipment and their wrappers) should be immediately taken out of service and impounded. These items should not be returned to the manufacturer (Darwin Professional Underwriters, Inc., 2006).

Incident Reporting

Incident or adverse event reporting should be utilized as a method to immediately document information about actual or potential injury to a patient, visitors, or staff. Despite limited research specifically on adverse events and potential adverse events in ambulatory care, studies suggest they may occur frequently and they may be quite different than those that occur in hospitals (Plews-Ogan et al., 2004).

It is management's responsibility to take action to prevent incident recurrence. It is important that all staff members know and practice the ambulatory center's policy and procedures for reporting incidents. That policy should define what is considered an incident; explain what should be done after an incident has occurred; designate who has responsibility for completing the report; and provide instruction on how paperwork should be completed. The facility's incident report forms should be composed in language appropriate to the particular state's peer review or quality assurance mandates in order to assure the greatest evidentiary protection (Darwin Professional Underwriters, Inc., 2006).

Sentinel Events

As part of its goal of enhancing patient safety and improving health care for the public, The Joint Commission has included as part of their accreditation process a review of organizations' responses to sentinel events. The Joint Commission has established a reporting system and database of sentinel events, including an analysis of the root cause, or underlying factors, which if eliminated could reduce the risk of repetition. Individual states may have adverse event reporting criteria and critical analysis that take precedence. Facility administrators should be fully versed in the protective aspects legislated by the state (Radtke, 2004).

The Joint Commission defines a sentinel event as "An unexpected occurrence involving death or serious physical or psychologic injury, or the risk thereof" (The Joint Commission, 2007). The term sentinel is used because it denotes the need for immediate attention and investigation. Sentinel events are not necessarily the same as medical errors;

sentinel events are not always caused by medical error, and errors may not become sentinel events. Serious injury includes loss of limb or function. Near miss events include occurrences and potential negative outcomes that almost happened. Identification and reporting of a sentinel event may result in The Joint Commission issuing a sentinel event alert to hospitals, ambulatory facilities, home care agencies, nursing homes, and behavioral health care institutions as appropriate, particularly if multiple similar events are reported. A sentinel event alert database, available online, supplies detailed information and the underlying cause of each event. Examples of past sentinel event alert topics include operating room fire, magnetic resonance imaging safety, operative site identification and pediatric medication errors. The full list and alerts can be accessed at www.jointcommission.com. The Joint Commission accredited facilities are expected to review alerts, assess their own processes against the alert recommendations and make appropriate changes to prevent future similar occurrences.

When a sentinel or adverse event occurs, root cause analysis should be utilized to identify why it happened, rather than just how it occurred (McDonald & Leyhane, 2005). The aim of root cause analysis is to identify process and system factors that, with appropriate changes, may reduce the risk of adverse patient outcomes (Radtke, 2004). Root cause analysis requires investigation by a multidisciplinary team that includes staff members with appropriate expertise and persons with decision-making authority using a predefined methodology that investigates and evaluates all possible contributing factors.

However, litigation of adverse events tends to be directed toward individual liability (Gosbee & Anderson, 2006). Thus, investigative teams also tend to focus on policy violations and personnel errors rather than underlying design-related factors. A shift in mind-set to adopting a systems-oriented perspective is essential. Understanding that many interdependent factors are involved in an event and that individual factors may have either positive or negative influence is vital to unbiased evaluation (Gosbee & Anderson, 2006). The root cause analysis team should avoid broad causal classification such as human error, equipment failure, or external factors because these factors are not isolated from potentially preventive measures (McDonald & Leyhane, 2006). Why the event happened as well as what happened and how it happened must be established.

When the team has identified necessary changes and developed a plan of action, it must be presented to senior management for approval and implementation, including long-term monitoring. Among the most difficult areas to improve are human factors, such as attention, memory, and the effects of interruptions (McDonald & Leyhane, 2006). The four major types of events are patient suicide (14%), wrong-site surgery (12.5%), operative and postoperative complications (12.3%), and medication errors (11%) (McDonald & Anderson, 2006).

MEDICATION SAFETY

Medication Errors

The derogatory effects of interruptions are especially applicable to medication errors. Nurses are subjected to many, and often unjustified, distractions and interruptions that affect working memory and the ability to focus at critical times (Pape et al., 2005). One out of five medications administered in hospitals and skilled nursing facilities is in error, while nearly 34% of preventable adverse drug events can be traced to the administrative process (Ketchum, Grass, & Padwojski, 2005).

Three important steps for the safe administration of medications are: verification of the patient's medical history; clarification of medication's appropriateness for the patient; reconciliation to resolve any discrepancies or changes in orders (Manno & Hayes, 2006). Because nontechnical forms and checklists requiring signatures have been shown to be effective in reducing medical errors, the facility should consider developing forms to be used by staff. The Institute for Healthcare Improvement (IHI) (www.ihi.org) and the Massachusetts Coalition for the Prevention of Medical Errors (www.macoalition.org) offer standardized forms and tool kits for developing medication reconciliation policies on their Web sites.

Medications that look or sound alike should be identified and a plan implemented to avoid errors in their use. For example, two medications with similar names could be addressed by purchasing a different brand of one with a name that is not so similar such as adrenalin instead of epinephrine to avoid mixing the latter up with ephedrine. National patient safety goals are now focusing on the potential for patient injury related to inappropriate use of anticoagulants in the perioperative time frame. Local anesthetic agents with and without epinephrine are another concern; they should be stored separately and well labeled to avoid confusion.

Medication Reconciliation

The IHI defines medical reconciliation as creating the most accurate possible list of all medications a patient is taking, including the details of administration, and comparing that list to the physician's admission, transfer, and/or discharge orders. The goal is to provide correct medications at all transition points during patient care – often the times of greatest error. New technologies include automated medication dispensing systems and computerized physician order entry; however, medication reconciliation reduces error regardless of technology or special equipment use (Ketchum, Grass, & Padwojski, 2005).

Since January 2006, all Joint Commission accredited facilities must have protocols for documenting and reconciling medications throughout the continuum of care (Manno & Hayes, 2006). Failing to reconcile medications may result in omitted doses, incorrect doses, incorrect route of administration, incorrect timing, and failure to stop discontinued drugs. Duplication of medications may occur with the use of generic and brand names for a single medication. Sixty percent of medication errors occur because of inadequate communication around transition points such as admission, transfer, and on discharge (Barnsteiner, 2005; Ketchum, Grass, & Padwojski, 2005; Vira, Colquhoun, & Etchellis, 2006).

Nursing Considerations

Staff education and awareness are especially important in controlling risks and should be frequently addressed in staff meetings and through continuing education efforts. The best prevention of injury and liability is having staff members who consider risk management a constant part of their duties. Prevention is the key to risk management.

Unexpected events and complications may occur as a result of human error, periods of reduced observation, environmental factors (e.g., inadequate lighting, limited patient access), poor communication, haste, and lack of preparation (Kost, 2004). Allegations frequently made against nurses include:

- failure to follow nursing protocols
- inadequate monitoring or observation of the patient
- administration of improper medications
- failure to follow current physician orders properly and promptly
- inappropriate intervention
- insufficient patient protection against injury, such as falls or burns.

It should be noted that a nurse may also be found negligent if he or she carries out an order that is unsafe or erroneous. Questionable orders should be clarified by the physician who wrote the order. Illegibility is a major concern. If the nurse is not familiar with the medication, dosage, or method of administration, he or she is responsible for contacting her supervisor or the physician who wrote the order for clarification. The nurse is expected to exercise prudent judgment at all times.

In an ambulatory setting, a study of medication errors and reconciliation found that if a discrepancy was found and the nurse asked the physician whether he or she wanted to makes changes, 94% of those orders were changed by the physician (Barnsteiner, 2005).

As discussed in previous chapters, meticulous documentation is necessary to prove actions taken and disprove allegations. Perioperative documentation is especially critical because of the need for frequent nursing interventions; the postanesthesia care unit (PACU) is recognized as a particularly vulnerable area for the nurse.

Documentation should be clear, concise, and objective, giving facts rather than subjective impressions. If a flowchart is being used and there is inadequate space, an addendum on a separate sheet should be used to chart all pertinent information.

Notes should never be written in the margins or between lines because such entries may appear to a jury as an attempt to alter the record. Similarly, if checklists and charting by exception are used, the exception or deviation from standards and expectations should be clearly explained in the exceptions column. An addendum may be attached for adequate description or clarification.

The use of abbreviations, acronyms, and symbols often result in misinterpretation of orders. Especially with medications, this misinterpretation may result in serious patient safety issues. Health facilities should establish approved abbreviations, acronyms, and symbols (American Hospital Association, 2005). Care should be taken to use only institution-approved abbreviations. The next caregiver must be able to correctly decipher these abbreviations. Standard abbreviations are also important if, years later, the nurse is asked to explain the documentation to a lay jury. Legally, errors in charting should not be obliterated; a line through the incorrect statement followed by the correct information is sufficient (Ireland, 1997).

The "Do Not Use" list of abbreviations presented in Table 8-1 was created by The Joint Commission as part of the requirements for meeting National Patient Safety Goal Requirements.

For information not charted at the correct time, a notation of "missed entry" should be made, followed by the information and time of occurrence. This documentation is expected to be done in a timely manner, not days or weeks later. Altering or making an addition at that late date constitutes tampering. In many states, tampering with a permanent record is considered a felony (Ireland, 1997).

Do not attach incident reports to the patient's chart or note that an incident report was completed. Document only the facts of the occurrence and response to the event, avoiding the term incident (Darwin Professional Underwriters, Inc., 2006).

If a patient is uncooperative, combative, or verbally abusive, this behavior should be documented. However, care must be taken to not use subjective descriptions or derogatory comments that could be interpreted as insensitive. It may be best to describe the patient's exact behavior so that any future reviewers may make their own interpretation of the happenings.

Minimizing the risk of incidental injury is an underemphasized management responsibility in the PACU (Mecca & Serrins, 1997). For example, it is management's responsibility to ensure that equipment is properly maintained and serviced on a regular, documented, schedule. They should set standards for the appropriate use of that equipment. Similarly, the appropriate use of bed rails, restraints, and other protective devices should be defined. Staffing levels and staff training must be well managed to ensure that appropriate coverage and levels of skill are available to deal with unfore-

TABLE 8-1: DO NOT USE LIST OF ABBREVIATIONS

The Joint Commission

Official "Do Not Use" List[1]

Do Not Use	Potential Problem	Use Instead
U (unit)	Mistaken for "0" (zero), the number "4" (four) or "cc"	Write "unit"
IU (International Unit)	Mistaken for IV (intravenous) or the number 10 (ten)	Write "International Unit"
Q.D., QD, q.d., qd (daily) Q.O.D., QOD, q.o.d, qod (every other day)	Mistaken for each other Period after the Q mistaken for "I" and the "O" mistaken for "I"	Write "daily" Write "every other day"
Trailing zero (X.0 mg)* Lack of leading zero (.X mg)	Decimal point is missed	Write X mg Write 0.X mg
MS MSO_4 and $MgSO_4$	Can mean morphine sulfate or magnesium sulfate Confused for one another	Write "morphine sulfate" Write "magnesium sulfate"

[1] Applies to all orders and all medication-related documentation that is handwritten (including free-text computer entry) or on pre-printed forms.

***Exception:** A "trailing zero" may be used only where required to demonstrate the level of precision of the value being reported, such as for laboratory results, imaging studies that report size of lesions, or catheter/tube sizes. It may not be used in medication orders or other medication-related documentation.

Additional Abbreviations, Acronyms and Symbols
(For possible future inclusion in the Official "Do Not Use" List)

Do Not Use	Potential Problem	Use Instead
> (greater than) < (less than)	Misinterpreted as the number "7" (seven) or the letter "L" Confused for one another	Write "greater than" Write "less than"
Abbreviations for drug names	Misinterpreted due to similar abbreviations for multiple drugs	Write drug names in full
Apothecary units	Unfamiliar to many practitioners Confused with metric units	Use metric units
@	Mistaken for the number "2" (two)	Write "at"
cc	Mistaken for U (units) when poorly written	Write "mL" or "ml" or "milliliters" ("mL" is preferred)
μg	Mistaken for mg (milligrams) resulting in one thousand-fold overdose	Write "mcg" or "micrograms"

Updated 3/5/09

seen clinical crises. Ideally, all nurses in the postoperative recovery area should have full PACU certification and the staffing ratios should never fall below accepted standards. If stringent staffing criteria are affected by cost constraints, management must guarantee that less skilled staff are appropriately supervised and that sufficient skilled personnel are always available to deal with worst-case events (Mecca & Serrins, 1997). Cross-training of staff to be efficient and capable in an area of care other than the one they normally practice in is both a risk management and cost-containment strategy that allows emergency staffing needs to be more easily managed.

Risk management and quality assurance programs can be carried out successfully only with the full cooperation of the staff. To encourage reporting of incidents or protocol deviations, the program must be nonthreatening and nonpunitive to the participants. These programs are meant to improve staff performance and should not be used as evaluations for promotion.

QUALITY IMPROVEMENT

Traditionally, delivering quality health care has meant providing care that meets the standards set by accrediting bodies such as The Joint Commission, Accreditation Association for Ambulatory Health Care (AAAHC), and state and federal agencies. Quality assurance (QA) referred to meeting these standards.

Currently, QA is usually linked with quality improvement, continuous quality improvement (CQI), or total quality management (TQM), with the intention of surpassing basic requirements and continually upgrading service and care. Clinical pathways, or predetermined care plans, may be considered variations of TQM. Their flowchart format produces standardized, concise care delivery plans with concomitant data tracking for specific procedures or diagnoses.

QA can be traced back over 150 years, when Florence Nightingale collected data that documented wounded and ill British soldiers admitted to field hospitals during the Crimean War, nearly one half of whom died. Her data so alarmed the military that steps were instituted to improve hygiene and medical and nursing care. Later, she quantitatively assessed mortality rates in a London hospital that resulted in serious inquiries regarding the effect of hospital care on mortality (Remensnyder, 1998).

Before World War I, Ernest Avery Codman, at the Massachusetts General Hospital, developed a method of assessing outcomes of treatment with detailed records. In 1917, the American College of Surgeons (ACS) established the Hospital Standardization Program, which has evolved through the efforts of physician organizations, culminating in the creation of the Joint Commission on Accreditation of Healthcare Organizations (JCAHO), now The Joint Commission (Remensnyder, 1998). Ambulatory care and facilities have only recently received formal QA attention, and quality improvement (QI) protocols are continually being revised due to changes in accreditation policies by governmental, professional, and consumer agencies.

The Joint Commission accreditation process emphasizes the following five areas of quality improvement designed to promote continuous quality improvement: leadership responsibility for quality improvement, techniques of quality improvement, education and training, communication and collaboration, and evaluation of effectiveness of QI activities. Additionally, there are nine dimensions of quality that can determine how a health care organization's functions may affect patients

These nine dimensions may be categorized into two concepts: (1) doing what's right and (2) doing it well. Doing the right thing encompasses efficacy and appropriateness of the care or intervention. Doing the right thing well involves availability of supplies and services; timeliness of care and services; methods of care and service delivery; continuity of care; safety of procedures, interventions, and environment; efficiency of the relationship between outcomes of care and the resources allocated; and the least-tangible aspects, respect and caring. The American Society of PeriAnesthesia Nurses' position on patient safety (Table 8-2) involves the core values of communication, advocacy, competency, efficiency, timeliness, and teamwork.

The concepts of QI are based largely on industrial models developed after World War II. Health care facilities share several characteristics of industrial QI. For example, the leadership of organizations drives the QI process; customer-supplier relationships are developed; leadership concentrates QI on variations in normal processes and seeks to control them; all organizational personnel are involved in the examining processes; and formal problem-solving methods and statistical tools are used (Remensnyder, 1998). Similarly, crew resource management (CRM) is an aviation industry tool being introduced in health care organizations because it focuses on communication and safety. The industry found that 70% of commercial flight accidents were caused by human error, and 56% of those involved failed communication among crew members. The CRM model

TABLE 8-2: A POSITION STATEMENT ON PERIANESTHESIA SAFETY

Position

The American Society of PeriAnesthesia Nurses (ASPAN) is highly committed as an advocate for a culture of safety in all perianesthesia practice settings. ASPAN's core values for the culture of safety include communication, advocacy, competency, efficiency, timeliness, and teamwork. Characteristics of this culture of safety delivered in an environment of caring and guided by principles of research and evidence-based practices, include but are not limited to:

1. Communication
   a. Reporting errors/unsafe practices
   b. Ensuring a complete and systematic approach to hand off processes and transfer of care
   c. Developing and using effective listening skills
2. Advocacy
   a. Protecting the patient from harm
   b. Upholding ethics of care
   c. Maintaining patients' rights
   d. Seeking and implementing best practices
3. Competency
   a. Achieving and supporting professional competence and competency building in clinical practice
   b. Initiating, supporting and providing education for staff and patients
   c. Demonstrating appropriate clinical judgment and critical thinking
   d. Measuring and monitoring quality measures and nurse sensitive indicators
4. Efficiency/Timeliness
   a. Maintaining a healthy environment of care
   b. Providing timely interventions and reports
   c. Appreciating cues and initiating appropriate interventions
5. Teamwork
   a. Collaborating with health care providers
   b. Building mutual respect and trust between all health care providers
   c. Supporting an organizational culture of safety

focuses on team-oriented decision making and problem solving (The Joint Commission, 2006a).

Analysis of outcomes has been directed primarily at mortality, morbidity, and costs of a single institution. This type of research is increasingly being replaced by the use of statewide, national, and provider databases, and patient preference and satisfaction has become one of the most important measurable outcomes.

QA versus QI

The relationship of QA and QI is sequential because QA triggers QI, which in turn triggers CQI. Processes in health care involve people, so there is a constant opportunity to improve care and services. Nurses have an advantage in dealing with CQI because it builds on the familiar concept of the nursing process (Messner & Lewis, 1996). CQI focuses on important processes such as education, patient assessment, patient rights, and organizational ethics. However, it relies on statistical data for decision making that allows the focus to change from individual performance to process improvement that creates objectivity in improving quality.

The Joint Commission recommends a Ten-Step Process for monitoring and evaluating quality:

1. Assign responsibility.
2. Delineate scope of care and service.
3. Identify important aspects of care and service.
4. Identify indicators of such aspects.
5. Establish a means to trigger evaluation.
6. Collect and organize data.
7. Initiate evaluation.
8. Take actions to improve care and service.
9. Assess the effectiveness of actions and ensure that improvement is maintained.
10. Communicate results to relevant individuals and groups.

When step 10 of the process is instituted and the information has been communicated, feedback may identify additional areas that require moving back to step 6 and proceeding through step 10 again. These 10 steps of QA thus set in motion QI analysis and procedures, illustrating the relationship between assurance and improvement. QI protocols can be designed to study any aspect of the patient's ambulatory surgical experience. Study results and improvement ideas should be evaluated among all staff members so they can improve their personal performance, resulting in improved patient safety (Greco, 2006)

However, some factors unique to ambulatory care make evaluation and assurance of quality especially challenging. Outcomes are typically difficult to define because adverse events or complications that occur after discharge may go unreported; health care workers have less control over the patient and postoperative care so much relies on predischarge patient education; postoperative coordination of care among several providers in the ambulatory setting may be difficult to achieve; and less patient rapport may be established with the surgeon than occurs with inpatients. All of these factors may result in failure of patient compliance and follow-up, both of which are critical to defining outcomes and assessing quality of care (Remensnyder, 1998). Nonetheless, an ambulatory surgical facility should make every effort to monitor performance by collecting data from patients concerning their postoperative course and their opinions of the facility and the care they received.

Nursing Considerations

Increasingly, facilities are being assessed across the entire organization rather than as separate departments (e.g., the nursing department); therefore, the importance of teamwork and cooperation cannot be underestimated. Staff involvement is essential. When staff members participate, they have a greater interest and investment in CQI (Messner & Lewis, 1996). All staff members should have the opportunity to participate in the development and implementation of a CQI program. Hands-on providers are closely involved with, and aware of, quality issues. Therefore, staff members should be involved in decision making.

A clinical team's ability to safely deliver quality patient care requires effective communication and interaction. Disruptive behavior from all levels of responsibility – physicians, nurses, and administrators – can prevent collaboration, affecting patient safety and working relationships. The American Medical Association considers disruptive behavior to be "personal behavior, whether verbal or physical, that affects or that potentially may affect patient care negatively" (AMA Code of Medical Ethics, E-9.045). That is, disruptive behavior is any behavior that interferes with good safe patient care. Disruptive behavior may be covert or overt, and includes remarks that undermine a coworker professionally.

Unfortunately, the most common behaviors fall into three main categories.

- Physical intimidation and violence – such as throwing objects, tantrums, or yelling directly into someone's face.
- Abusiveness – usually expressed verbally by sarcastic or demeaning remarks.
- Refusal to cooperate – including refusal to follow directives, accept group decisions, or accept input

(The Joint Commission, 2006b)

Establishing a cooperative organizational culture is largely dependent on a zero-tolerance policy, preferably developed by staff and management and enforced by persons in leadership portions. A plausible strategy may be to include and discuss the zero-tolerance strategy as part of orientation and education (The Joint Commission, 2006b).

Staff education and CQI training are essential for a viable, ongoing program. QI and CQI efforts take time to implement and integrate; ten years is often the projection. Without the ongoing support and cooperation of the staff, success is unlikely.

SUMMARY

The primary goals of an ambulatory surgical center are patient safety and satisfaction. Risk management and quality monitoring are essential to accomplishing these goals. In order for the facility to establish and maintain an optimal level of quality care, staff members must know the level of performance expected of them and how best to continually provide it. Teamwork is essential for an ambulatory surgical center to be able to provide quality care that results in patient safety and satisfaction.

EXAM QUESTIONS

CHAPTER 8
Questions 97-100

Note: Choose the option that BEST answers each question.

97. One of the most important measurable outcomes of quality assurance (QA) and quality improvement (QI) programs is

    a. staff participation.
    b. patient satisfaction.
    c. cost containment.
    d. protocol designation.

98. If there is insufficient room for adequate charting, the nurse should

    a. restrict documentation to highlights.
    b. write in the margin and initial the notation.
    c. insert information between lines at the appropriate time interval.
    d. attach an addendum with full documentation.

99. An important management responsibility for patient safety is

    a. data retrieval.
    b. cost containment.
    c. maintenance of equipment.
    d. staff manipulation.

100. The Joint Commission evolved from the

    a. American Hospital Association Initiative.
    b. American Society of Anesthesiologists Position Paper.
    c. American College of Physicians Directive.
    d. Hospital Standardization Program.

This concludes the final examination.
Please answer the evaluation questions found on page v of this workbook.

RESOURCES

SUGGESTED READING

Association of periOperative Registered Nurses. (2005, April). AORN position statement on care of the perioperative patient with an implanted electronic device. Retrieved April 28, 2009, from http://www.aorn.org/PracticeResources/AORNPositionStatements/Position_IED/

Bragg, K., VanBalen, N., & Cook, N. (2005). Future trends in minimally invasive surgery. *AORN Journal, 82*(6), 105-118.

Gordon, D.B., Dahl, J., Pillips, P., Frandsen, J., Cowley, C., Foster, R., Fine, P., Miascowski, C., Fishman, S., & Finley, R. (2005). The use of as-needed range orders for opioid analgesics in the management of acute pain: A consensus statement of the American Society for Pain Management Nursing and the American Pain Society. *Home Healthcare Nurse, 23*(6), 388-96.

The Joint Commission. (2008, October). *2009 national patient safety goals ambulatory care program.* Retrieved April 25, 2009, from http://www.jointcommission.org/PatientSafety/NationalPatientSafetyGoals/09_amb_npsgs.htm

Mamaril, M.E., Ross, J.M., Krenzischek, D., O'Brien, D., Wilson, L. Clark, M., Clifford, T., & Hooper, V. (2006). The ASPAN's EBP conceptual model: Framework for perianesthesia and research. *Journal of Perianesthesia Nursing, 21*(3), 157-167.

O'Connell, M.P. (2006). Position impact on the surgical patient. *Nursing Clinics of North America, 41,* 173-192.

Watt-Watson, J., Chung, F., Chan, V.W., & McGillion, M. (2004). Pain management following discharge after ambulatory same-day surgery. *Journal of Nursing Management, 12*(3), 153-161.

Wilford Holm, S., Cunningham, L.L., Bensadoun, E., & Madsen, M. (2006). Hypertenision: Classification, pathophysiology, and management during outpatient sedation and local anesthesia. *Journal of Oral and Maxillary Surgery, 64*(1), 111-121.

GLOSSARY

agonist: A pharmacologic agent that has affinity and efficacy and interacts with receptors to produce a response.

analgesia: Reduction of pain perception.

anesthesia: Loss of feeling or sensation; frequently used to refer to insensibility to pain.

anoxia: Reduction of oxygen in body tissues below physiologic levels.

antagonist: An agent that nullifies the action of another agent.

antibody: Complex molecule (immunoglobulin) produced by the lymph system in response to an antigen.

anticholinergics: Pharmacologic agents that block the effects of parasympathetic nerves.

antigen: A chemical substance or small organism whose entry into the body provokes an immune system response and the formation of an antibody or immunoglobulin.

antisialagogue: A drug that inhibits excessive salivary secretion.

anxiolytics: Pharmacologic agents that reduce anxiety and nervous excitement.

apnea: A cessation of breathing; the absence of respiration.

arteriosclerosis: Thickening, hardening, and loss of elasticity of the arterial walls.

ASA physical status: A classification system developed by the American Society of Anesthesiologists that ranks viable patients from P1 to P5, with ascending numbers indicating increasing risk of morbidity and mortality during surgery and anesthesia.

aspiration: Inhalation of foreign material into the respiratory passages.

atelectasis: Collapse of alveolar sacs in the lungs.

atherosclerosis: An accumulation of fatty deposits (plaque) along the interior walls of large- and medium-sized arteries.

benzodiazepines: A group of pharmacologic agents that produce dose-related sedation, anxiolysis, and amnesia. Minor tranquilizers.

bronchospasm: A severe constriction of the bronchial tree.

butyrophenones: A group of major tranquilizers pharmacologically and clinically similar to phenothiazines.

capnography: Measurement of carbon dioxide tension or content in exhaled breath using infrared light technology.

credentials: Professional credentials of a practitioner regarding education, training, experience, and performance.

dermatome: An area of the body that is innervated from one spinal root.

dysphoria: Restlessness, agitation, exaggerated feelings.

dysrhythmia: A disturbance of rhythm.

embolus: A single mass of tissue, fat, clotted blood, or a bubble of air or gas that is traveling through the circulatory system.

endoscopy: Visualization of the interior of a body cavity using a lighted instrument.

endotracheal intubation: Insertion of a specialized tube through the nasopharynx or oropharynx and between the vocal cords into the trachea to establish a controllable, patent airway.

epidural anesthesia: Loss of sensation produced by the injection of a local anesthetic outside the dura mater but within the spinal canal.

general anesthesia: Pharmacologically induced unconsciousness and insensibility to pain.

hypercapnia/hypercarbia: Excessive amount of carbon dioxide in the blood; a carbon dioxide pressure greater than 45 to 50 torr.

hyperkalemia: Excessive amount of potassium in the blood.

hyperpnea: Increased depth of respiration.

hyperventilation: An increased rate and depth of breathing, resulting in an abnormal lowering in arterial carbon dioxide content.

hypnotics: Pharmacologic agents that can produce a state of central nervous system depression similar to sleep.

hypocapnia/hypocarbia: Subnormal amount of carbon dioxide in the blood.

hyponatremia: Decreased concentration of sodium in the blood.

hypopharynx (laryngopharynx): Lowest portion of the pharynx, leading to the larynx and esophagus.

hypothermia: Low body temperature.

hypoventilation: Reduced rate and depth of breathing, resulting in a decrease in arterial oxygen content and increase in carbon dioxide content.

hypovolemia: Decreased circulating blood volume.

hypoxemia: An inadequate oxygen supply in the blood; an arterial oxygen pressure of less than 60 torr.

hypoxia: Reduced oxygen content or tension, as in inspired air or body tissues.

inhalation anesthesia: A state of general anesthesia produced by inhalation of a vaporized volatile liquid anesthetic or gaseous anesthetic.

ischemia: Localized deficiency of blood supply, chiefly due to contraction or obstruction of a blood vessel.

laparoscopy: Endoscopic examination of the interior of the abdomen by means of a laparoscope.

laryngospasm: A severe constriction of the larynx.

larynx: The organ of voice production. A musculocartilaginous structure located at the top of the trachea, below the base of the tongue, anterior to the esophagus, and covered by the epiglottis during swallowing.

local anesthetic: An agent whose anesthetic action is limited to an area of the body determined by the site of injection or application.

monitoring: Clinical assessment by direct observation or mechanical devices.

neuromuscular blocking agents: Pharmacologic agents that block transmission of impulses at the neuromuscular junction, causing paralysis of striated muscles.

opioid: Any agonist drug with morphine-like activity.

orthostatic hypotension: A fall in blood pressure, associated with dizziness, that occurs upon standing or sitting upright.

oximetry: Photoelectronic measurement of the oxygen saturation of arterial blood.

pharmacokinetic: Relating to the time course of a drug and its metabolites in the body after administration by any route.

pharynx: The portion of the airway between the nasal cavity and the larynx; consists of the nasopharynx, oropharynx, and hypopharynx (laryngopharynx). Commonly referred to as the throat.

phenothiazines: A group of potent tranquilizers with antipsychotic action that often also exhibit antiemetic and antihistaminic effect.

pneumonitis: Inflammation of the lung.

pneumothorax: An accumulation of air or gas in the pleural cavity; results in a progressive increase in intrapleural pressure with lung collapse and impairment of circulation.

procedural sedation/analgesia: A state of minimally depressed consciousness in which the patient independently maintains airway control and responds appropriately to physical stimulation and verbal command.

prophylaxis: Prevention or protection against occurrence, injury, or disease.

proprioception: Awareness of movement and position.

pruritus: Uncomfortable sensation of the skin leading to the urge to scratch.

rales: Abnormal breath sounds produced by the flow of air through alveoli and bronchioles that are constricted by spasm or filled with secretions.

regional anesthesia: Loss of sensation in a particular area of the body.

regurgitation: A backward flow, as with the flow of undigested food or gastric fluid into the esophagus.

rhonchi: Coarse, rattling sound usually caused by secretions in the bronchial tubes.

root cause analysis: A process of identifying the cause(s) of variation in performance.

sedatives: Drugs that promote calmness and drowsiness and may produce some degree of amnesia and altered time perception.

somnolence: Prolonged or unnatural sleepiness or drowsiness.

spinal anesthesia: Loss of sensation and motor paralysis produced by the injection of a local anesthetic agent into the subarachnoid space around the spinal cord. Also referred to as subarachnoid or intrathecal anesthesia.

stridor: A harsh, high-pitched respiratory sound associated with severe upper-airway obstruction.

tachypnea: Excessively rapid rate of respiration (over 25 breaths per minute in adults).

trachea: The cartilaginous tube extending from the larynx to its division into the mainstem bronchi.

vasopressor: An agent that produces systemic arterial vasoconstriction resulting in a rise in blood pressure.

wheeze: A high-pitched, whistling sound characterizing an obstruction or spasm of the lower airways.

BIBLIOGRAPHY

Accreditation Association for Ambulatory Health Care, Inc. (2007). *Accreditation laws and regulations by state.* Retrieved April 27, 2009, from http//:www.aaahc.org/lawsbystate.htm

Accreditation Association for Ambulatory Health Care, Inc. (2006). *New York Law: Fact sheets.* Retrieved April 27, 2009, from http://www.aaahcnewyork.org/factsheets.htm

Accreditation Association for Ambulatory Health Care, Inc. (1998, September). AAAHC Update. Skokie, IL: Author.

Aker, J. (2001). Safety of ambulatory surgery. *Journal of PeriAnesthesia Nursing, 16*(6), 353-358.

Ambulatory Surgery Center Association. (n.d.-a). *Frequently asked questions about ambulatory surgery centers.* Retrieved October 11, 2007, from http://www.ascassociation.org/faqs/faqaboutascs/

Ambulatory Surgery Center Association. (n.d.-b). *Meeting America's surgical needs.* [Brochure] Retrieved April 26, 2009, from http://www.ascassociation.org/masn.pdf

Ambulatory Surgery Center Association. (n.d.-c). *The history of ACSs.* Retrieved October 11, 2007, from http://www.ascassociation.org/faqs/aschistory/

American Academy of Ambulatory Care Nursing. (2006). Membership brochure. Available at http//:www.aaacn.org/membership/membership_brochure.pdf

American Association for Accreditation of Ambulatory Surgery Facilities, Inc. (2006). *For consumers.* Retrieved April 27, 2009, from http//:www .aaaasf.org/consumers.php

American Association for Accreditation of Ambulatory Surgery Facilities, Inc. (1998). *Background.* Mundelein, IL: Author.

American Association of Nurse Anesthetists. (2003, June). *Considerations for policy guidelines for registered nurses engaged in the administration of sedation and analgesia.* Retrieved April 27, 2009, from http://www.aana.com/Resources.aspx

American Association of Nurse Anesthetists. (2001). *AANA latex protocol.* Retrieved October 11, 2007, from http://www.aana.com/resources.aspx?ucNavMenu_TSMenuTargetID=51&ucNavMenu_TSMenuTargetType=4&ucNavMenu_TSMenuID=6&id=765

American Board of Perianesthesia Nursing Certification. (n.d.). *About Us.* Retrieved February 1, 2007, from http://www.cpancapa.org/about/index/htm

American College of Surgeons. (2006). *Surgical care improvement project (SCIP).* Retrieved October 15, 2007, from http://www.facs.org/cqi/scip.html

American College of Surgeons. (n.d.). *Giving your informed consent.* Retrieved February 1, 2007, from http://www.facs.org/public_info/operation/consent.html

American Hospital Association. (2005). *Hospital Health Network, 79*(6), 41-42.

American Society of Anesthesiologists. (2005). *Natural rubber latex allergy: Considerations for anesthesiologists*. Retrieved April 27, 2009, from http://asahq.org/publication&Services/latex allergy.pdf

American Society of Anesthesiologists. (2004, October 27). *Excerpted from continuum of depth of sedation definition of general anesthesia and levels of sedation/analgesia*. Retrieved September 20, 2007, from http://www.asahq.org/publicationsAndServices/standards/20.pdf

American Society of Anesthesiologists. (2002). Practice guidelines for sedation and analgesia for non-anesthesiologists. *Anesthesiology, 96*(4), 1004-1007.

American Society of Anesthesiologists. (1998). *Relative value guide*. Park Ridge, IL: Author.

American Society of PeriAnesthesia Nurses. (1996, November 12). *A position statement on perianesthesia advanced practice nursing*. Retrieved May 5, 2009, from http://www.aspan.org/ClinicalPractice/PositionStatements/tabid/3253/Default.aspx

American Society of PeriAnesthesia Nurses. (1998). *Standards of perianesthesia nursing practice*. Thorofare, NJ: Author.

American Society of PeriAnesthesia Nurses. (1999, April 18). *A position statement on fast tracking*. Retrieved May 5, 2009, from http://www.aspan.org/ClinicalPractice/PositionStatements/tabid/3253/Default.aspx

American Society of PeriAnesthesia Nurses. (2003, April 3). *A position statement on visitation in phase I level care*. Retrieved May 5, 2009, from http://www.aspan.org/ClinicalPractice/PositionStatements/tabid/3253/Default.aspx

Anderson, L.G. (1997). Ambulatory care. In J. M. Black & E. Matassarian-Jacobs (Eds.), *Medical-surgical nursing: Clinical management for continuity of care* (5th ed., pp. 135-142). Philadelphia: W.B. Saunders Company.

Ang-Lee, M., Yuan, C.S., & Moss, J. (2005). Complementary and alternative therapies. In R. Miller (Ed.), *Miller's Anesthesia* (6th ed., pp. 1653-1684). Philadelphia: Elsevier Churchill Livingstone.

Association of Operating Room Nurses, Inc. (2006). *Recommended practices for managing the patient receiving conscious sedation/analgesia*. AORN Standards, Recommended Practices, and Guidelines. Denver, CO: Author.

AstraZeneca Pharmaceuticals. (2005). Deprivan 1% package insert. Accessed June 10, 2009, from http://www1.astrazeneca-us.com/pi/deprivan.pdf

Bachenberg, K. (2005). Issues of outpatient surgery and obstructive sleep apnea. *Newsletter of the Society for Ambulatory Anesthesia: Ambulatory Anesthesia, 20*(3), 6-7. Accessed June 22, 2009, from http://www.sambahq.org/professional-info/newsletter/July2005.pdf

Baker, K. & Landriscina, D. (2007). The Icarus effect: The influence of dilutent warming on dantolene sodium mixing time. *AANA Journal, 75,* 101-106.

Barnett, S.R. (2001). Ambulatory anesthesia for the elderly: Grandma on the move. *Ambulatory Anesthesia, 16*(2), 5-6.

Barnes, S. & O'Brien, D. (2002). Considering bypass of phase I PACU? *Journal of Perianesthesia Nursing, 17*(5), 193-195.

Barnsteiner, J.H. (2005). Medication reconciliation: Transfer of medication information across settings – keeping it free from error. *Journal of Infusion Nursing, 28,* 31-36.

Belani, K.G. (2003). Ketorolac: A choice pediatric drugs, with some limitations. *Ambulatory Anesthesia, 18*(2), 3-4.

Belani, K.G. (2005). Postanesthetic shivering and treatment options: An overview. *Ambulatory Anesthesia, 20*(1), 8-9.

Bernstein, M. (1996). An overview of latex allergy and its implications for emergency nurses. *Journal of Emergency Nursing, 22,* 29-36.

Berrio, M.W. & Levesque, M.E. (1996). Advance directives. Most patients don't have one. Do yours? *American Journal of Nursing, 96,* 25-28.

Brandom, B.W. (2005). The genetics of malignant hyperthermia. *Anesthesiology Clinics of North America, 23,* 615-619.

Brislin, R.P. & Rose, J.B. (2005). Pediatric acute pain management. *Anesthesiology Clinics of North America, 23,* 789-814.

Brockway, P.M. (1997). The ambulatory nurse: Evolution, competency, and vision. *Nursing Clinics of North America, 32*(2), 387-394.

Brown, D.L. (2005). Spinal, epidural, and caudal. In R. Miller (Ed.), *Miller's Anesthesia* (6th ed. pp. 1653-1684). Philadelphia: Elsevier Churchill Livingstone.

Brown, K. (2005). Pediatric obstructive sleep apnea and obesity, *Newsletter of the Society for Ambulatory Anesthesia: Ambulatory Anesthesia, 20*(3), 7-8. Accessed June 22, 2009, from http://www.sambahq .org/professional-info/newsletter/July2005.pdf

Brown, M. (1997). Neuromuscular blockade. In M. Brown & E.M. Brown (Eds.), *Comprehensive postanesthesia care* (pp. 105-116). Baltimore: Williams & Wilkins.

Brown, O.W. (1997). Surgical considerations. In M. Brown & E.M. Brown (Eds.), *Comprehensive postanesthesia care* (pp. 483-487). Baltimore: Williams & Wilkins.

Bumgarner, S.D. & Evans, M.L. (1999). Clinical care map for the ambulatory laparoscopic cholecystectomy patient. *Journal of PeriAnesthesia Nursing, 14*(1), 12-16.

Burden, N. (2000). The specialty of ambulatory surgery. In N. Burden (Ed.), *Ambulatory surgical nursing* (2nd ed., pp. 3-22). Philadelphia: W.B. Saunders.

Burden, N. (2004). Discharge planning for the elderly ambulatory surgical patient. *Journal of PeriAnesthesia Nursing, 19*(6), 401-405.

Burns, L.J. (1996). Intraoperative nursing and anesthesia. In S.C. Smeltzer & B.G. Bare (Eds.), *Brunner and Suddarth's textbook of medical-surgical nursing* (8th ed., p. 377). Philadelphia: Lippincott-Raven.

Centers for Medicare and Medicaid Service. (2009). *Revised Appendix L, Interpretive Guidelines for Ambulatory Surgical Centers.* Accessed June 15, 2009, from http:// ascassociation.org//guidelines.pdf

Chung, D.C. & Lam, A.M. (1997). *Essentials of anesthesiology* (3rd ed.). Philadelphia: W.B. Saunders Company.

Cleveland Clinic. (2006). *Allergy overview.* Retrieved April 26, 2009, from http://www .clevelandclinic.org/disorders/allergies/pul_overview.aspx

Clifford, T.L., Mamaril, M., & Sullivan, E. (2005). The history of ASPAN standards. *Journal of PeriAnesthesia Nursing, 20*(6), 380-384.

Cohn, J.C., Klinger, P.J., & Hinder, R.A. (1997). Laparoscopic Nissen fundoplication as an ambulatory surgery center procedure. *Today's Surgical Nurse, 19*(4), 27-30.

Coll, A. & Ameen, J. (2006). Profiles of pain after day surgery: Patients' experiences of three different operation types. *Journal of Advanced Nursing, 53*(2), 176-184.

Coll, A., Ameen, J., & Mosely L. (2004). Reported pain after day surgery: A critical literature review. *Journal of Advanced Nursing, 46*(1), 53-65.

Conahan, T.J. & Young, M.L. (1997). Outpatient anesthesia. In D.E. Longnecker & F.L. Murphy (Eds.), *Introduction to anesthesia* (9th ed., pp. 377-385). Philadelphia: W.B. Saunders Company.

Connor, R. & Fogg, D. (Eds.). (1999). *Ambulatory surgical principles and practices.* Denver: Association of Operating Room Nurses, Inc.

Cook, F. & Rooke, R. (2003). Priorities in perioperative geriatrics. *Anesthesia & Analgesia, 9,* 1823-1836.

Cowling, G.E. & Haas, R.E. (2002). Hypotension in the PACU: An algorithmic approach. *Journal of PeriAnesthesia Nursing, 17*(3), 159-163.

Cote, C.J. (2002). Preparation, premedication, and induction of anesthesia in children. *Ambulatory Anesthesia, 17*(1), 5-6.

Cote, C.J. (2005). Pediatric anesthesia. In R. Miller, (Ed.), *Miller's anesthesia* (6th ed.), Philadelphia: Elsevier Churchill Livingstone.

D'Amours, D.H. (1997). Nerve blocks. In D.E. Longnecker & F.L. Murphy (Eds.), *Introduction to anesthesia* (9th ed., pp. 201-215). Philadelphia: W.B. Saunders Company.

Darwin Professional Underwriters, Inc. (2006, October 23). Incident reporting: Fast-tracking information, nothing more, nothing less? *Today's Surgicenter.* Retrieved June 11, 2009, from http://www.surgistrategies.com/articles/6a1feat1.html

Dershwitz, M. (1998). Agents for general anesthesia. In B.D. Schirmer & D.W. Rattner (Eds.), *Ambulatory surgery* (pp. 123-136). Philadelphia: W.B. Saunders Company.

DeFazio-Quinn, D.M. (1997). Ambulatory surgery: An evolution. *Nursing Clinics of North America, 32*(2), 377–386.

Dewar, A., Scott, J., & Muir, J. (2004). Telephone follow-up for day surgery patients: patient perceptions and nurses' experiences. *Journal of Perianesthesia Nursing, 19*(4), 234-241.

Donlon, J.V., Doyle, D.J, & Feldman, M.A. (2005). Anesthesia for eye, ear, nose, and throat surgery. In R. Miller (Ed.), *Miller's anesthesia* (6th ed.). Philadelphia: Elsevier Churchill Livingstone.

Dorian, R.S. (2005). Anesthesia. In F.C. Brunicardi, D.K. Anderson, T.R. Billiar, D.L. Dunn, J.G. Hunter, & R.G. Pollack (Eds.), *Schwartz's principles of surgery* (8th ed.). New York: McGraw Hill, Health Publishing Division.

Doyle, C.E. (1999). Preoperative strategies for managing postoperative pain at home after day surgery. *Journal of PeriAnesthesia Nursing, 14*(6), 373-379.

Drain, C.B. (2009). Care of the ear, nose, throat, neck and maxillofacial surgical patient. In C.B. Drain & J. Forren (Eds.), *Perianesthesia nursing: A critical care approach* (5th ed., pp. 458-475). St. Louis: Saunders Elsevier.

Dunn, D. (1998). Preoperative assessment criteria and patient teaching for ambulatory surgery patients. *Journal of PeriAnesthesia Nursing, 13*(5), 274-291.

Drug Consult. (2006). Clinical Pharmacology, Gold Standard Multimedia.

Ead, H. (2006). From Aldrete to PADDS: Reviewing discharge criteria after ambulatory surgery. *Journal of PeriAnesthesia Nursing, 21*(4), 259-267.

Ebert, T.J., Shankar, H., & Haake, R. (2006). Perioperative consideration for patients with morbid obesity. *Anesthesiology Clinics of North America, 24,* 621-636.

Eckhardt, W.F. (1998). Local and regional anesthesia. In B.D. Schirmer & D.W. Rattner (Eds.), *Ambulatory surgery* (pp. 151-166). Philadelphia: W.B. Saunders Company.

Egan, T. (2001). In M. Vann, "Grandma Enters New Age: A Report from the ASA Annual Meeting." *Newsletter of the Society for Ambulatory Anesthesia: Ambulatory Anesthesia, 16*(2), 6. Accessed June 12, 2009, from http://www.sambahq.org/professional-info/newsletter/NewApril_2001.pdf

Eger, E.I. (2004). Characteristics of anesthetic agents used for induction and maintenance of general anesthesia, *American Journal of Health-System Pharmacists,* 61 Suppl. 4, 53-58.

Ellis, K. (2006, February 1). *Otolaryngology in ASCs: A growing frontier for technology.* Retrieved April 26, 2009, from http://www.vpico.com/articlemanager/printerfriendly.aspx?article=108314

Federated Ambulatory Surgery Association. (n.d.). *Recovery care.* Retrieved October 11, 2007.

Federated Ambulatory Surgery Association. (2007). *Letter to administrator, Center for Medicare and Medicaid Services, Oct. 30, 2007.* Accessed June 11, 2009, from http://www.fasa.org

Federated Ambulatory Surgery Association. (1996). *Recovery care survey.* Alexandria, VA: Author.

Federated Ambulatory Surgery Association. (1998). *Healthcare answers.* Alexandria, VA: Author.

The Federation of State Medical Boards. (2002). Report Of The Special Committee On Outpatient (Office-Based) Surgery. Accessed June 11, 2009, from http://www.fsmb.org/pdf/2002_grpol_Outpatient_Surgery.pdf

Fetzer, S.J., Hand, M.A., Bouchard, P.A., Smith, H.B., & Jenkins, M.B. (2005). Self-care activities for post discharge nausea and vomiting. *Journal of Perianesthesia Nursing, 20*(4), 249-254.

Fleisher, L.A., Yee, K., Lillemoe, K.D., Talami, M.A., Yeo, C.J., Heath, R., et al. (1999). Is outpatient laparoscopy safe and cost-effective? A model to study transition of care. *Anesthesiology, 90*(6), 1746-1755.

Fox, V.J. (1998). Postoperative education that works. *AORN Journal, 67*(5), 1010-1017.

Gaiser, R.R. (1997). Spinal, epidural, and caudal anesthesia. In D.E. Longnecker & F.L. Murphy (Eds.), *Introduction to anesthesia* (9th ed., pp. 216-231). Philadelphia: W.B. Saunders Company.

Geiger-Bronsky, M. (1998). Pulmonary rehabilitation and self-care after ambulatory surgery. *Journal of PeriAnesthesia Nursing, 13*(6), 382-393.

Golembiewski, J. (2006). Antidepressants: Pharmacology and implications in the perioperative period, *Journal of PeriAnesthesia Nursing, 21*(40), 285-87.

Gordon, D., Dahl, J., Pillips, P., Frandsen, J., Cowley, C., Foster, R., et al. (2005). The use of as-needed range orders for opioid analgesics in the management of acute pain: A consensus statement of the American Society for Pain Management Nursing and the American Pain Society. *Home Healthcare Nurse, 23*(6), 388-396.

Gosbee, J. & Anderson, T. (2003) Human factors engineering design demonstrations can enlighten your RCA team. *Quality and Safety in Health Care, 12,* 119-121.

Greco, R.J. (2006) Quality improvement: Implement error reduction practices to improve patient safety. *The ASF Source, Fall 2006,* 9-11.

Gronert, G.A., Pessah, I.N., Muldoon, S.M., & Taute, T.J. (2005). Malignant hyperthermia. In R. Miller (Ed.), *Miller's Anesthesia* (6th ed.). Philadelphia: Elsevier Churchill Livingstone.

Guida, B.A. (2004). The role of the nurse practitioner in an ambulatory surgery unit. *AORN, 79*(3), 606-615.

Hardin, R.E. & Zenilman, M.E. (2005). Surgical considerations in the elderly. In F.C. Brunicardi, D.K. Anderson, T.R. Billiar, D.L. Dunn, J.G. Hunter, & R.G. Pollack (Eds.), *Schwartz's principles of surgery* (8th ed.). New York: McGraw Hill, Health Publishing Division.

Hickok, C.B. & Weintraub, H.D. (1997). Special considerations for ambulatory surgical patients. In M. Brown & E.M. Brown (Eds.), *Comprehensive postanesthesia care* (pp. 468-481). Baltimore: Williams & Wilkins.

Horvath, K.J. (2003). Postoperative recovery at home after gynecolocgic laparoscopic surgery. *Journal of PeriAnesthesia Nursing, 18*(5), 324-334.

Hunter, J.J. (2005). Laparoscopic surgery. In F.C. Brunicardi, D.K. Anderson, T.R. Billiar, D.L. Dunn, J.G. Hunter, & R.G. Pollack (Eds.), *Schwartz's principles of surgery* (8th ed.). New York: McGraw Hill, Health Publishing Division.

Hwang, J.C.F., Bill, T.J., & Edlich, R.F. (1998). Preoperative assessment and discharge assessment criteria. In B.D. Schirmer & D.W. Rattner (Eds.), *Ambulatory surgery* (pp. 74-80). Philadelphia: W.B. Saunders Company.

Informed Health Choices. (2006). Results of National Study of ASCs. Available on-line: http://www.informedhc.com

Ireland, D. (1997). Legal issues in ambulatory surgery. *Nursing Clinics of North America, 32*(2), 469-476.

Ireland, D. (2006) Surgical concerns of pediatric patients. *Nursing Clinics of North America, 41,* 265-298.

Jablonka, D.H. & Davis, P.J. (2005). Opioids in pediatric anesthesia. *Anesthesiology Clinics of North America, 23,* 621-634.

Joint Commission on Accreditation of Healthcare Organizations. (1997). *A crosswalk between the American College of Surgeons' guidelines for optimal office-based surgery and the Joint Commission's ambulatory care standards.* Oakbrook, IL: Author.

Joshi, G.P. (2006). Are patients with obstructive sleep apnea syndrome suitable for ambulatory surgery? *ASA Newsletter, 70*(1).

Joshi, G.P. & Kehlet, H. (2006). A procedure specific approach to improve postoperative pain management. *ASA Newsletter, 70*(9).

Juarez, G., Cullinane, C.A., Borneman, T., Fatabella, A., Ferrell, B.R., Wagman, L.D., Lew, M. (2005). Management of pain and nausea in outpatient surgery. *Pain Management Nursing, 6*(4), 175-181.

Kamming, D. & Chung, F. (2004). What criteria should be used for discharge after outpatient surgery. In L. Fleisher (Ed.), *Evidence-based practice of anesthesiology* (pp. 247-252). Philadelphia: Saunders.

Kamming, D., Chung, F., Williams, D., McGrath, B., & Bruna, C. (2004). Pain management in ambulatory surgery. *Journal of PeriAnesthesia Nursing, 19*(3), 174-182.

Kankkunen, P., Vehvilainen-Julkunen, K., Pietila, A., & Halonen, P. (2003). Is the sufficiency of discharge instructions related to children's postoperative pain at home after day surgery? *Nordic College of Caring Sciences, Scandinavian Journal of Caring Sciences, 17,* 365-372.

Karlet, M.C. (1998). Malignant hyperthermia: Considerations for ambulatory surgery. *Journal of PeriAnesthesia Nursing, 13*(5), 304-312.

Keita, H., Benifla, J.L., Le Bouar, V., & Porcher, R. (2003). Prophylactic ip injection of bupivacaine and/or morphine does not improve postoperative analgesia after laparoscopic gynecologic surgery. *Canadian Journal of Anesthesia, 4,* 362-367.

Kennedy, S.K. (1997). Nonopioid intravenous anesthetics. In D.E. Longnecker & F.L. Murphy (Eds.), *Introduction to anesthesia* (9th ed., pp. 66-98). Philadelphia: W.B. Saunders Company.

Kervin, M.W. (2002). Residual neuromuscular blockade in the immediate portoperative period, *Journal of PeriAnesthesia Nursing, 17*(3), 151-158.

Ketchum, K., Grass, C.A., & Padwojski, A. (2005). *American Journal of Nursing, 105*(11), 78-85.

Kleinman, W. & Mikhail, M. (2006). Spinal, epidural, and caudal anesthesia. In G.E. Morgan, M.S. Mikhail, & M.J. Murray (Eds.), *Clinical anesthesiology* (4th ed., pp 289-323). New York: Mcgraw Hill.

Knoerl, D.V., McNulty, P., Estes, C., &Conley, K. (2001). Evaluation of orthostatic blood pressure testing as a discharge criterion from PACU after spinal anesthesia. *Journal of Perianesthesia Nursing, 16*(1), 11-18.

Kolcaba, K. & Wilson, L. (2002). Comfort care: A framework for perianesthesia nursing. *Journal of PeriAnesthesia Nursing, 17*(2), 102-114.

Kost, M. (2004). Moderate sedation/analgesia core competencies for practice. St. Louis:Saunders.

Kost, M. (2003). Administration of conscious sedation/analgesia. *Nursing Spectrum.* Retrieved April 24, 2009, from http://www.nursing specturm.com/ce/ cc159.htm

Kozar, R.A. & Moore, F.A. (2005). Fluids and electrolytes. In F.C. Brunicardi, D.K. Anderson, T.R. Billiar, D.L. Dunn, J.G. Hunter, & R.G. Pollack (Eds.), *Schwartz's principles of surgery* (8th Ed.). New York: McGraw Hill, Health Publishing Division.

Kramer, T.H. (1997). Opioids in anesthesia practice. In D.E. Longnecker & F.L. Murphy (Eds.), *Introduction to anesthesia* (9th ed., pp. 99-109). Philadelphia: W.B. Saunders Company.

Krechel, S.W. (1997). Special considerations in the geriatric population. In M. Brown & E.M. Brown (Eds.), *Comprehensive postanesthesia care* (pp. 409-433). Baltimore: Williams & Wilkins.

Lam, D., Miranda, R., & Hom, S.J. (1997). Laparoscopic cholecystectomy as an outpatient procedure. *Journal of the American College of Surgeons, 185,* 152-155.

Lancaster, K.A. (1997). Care of the pediatric patient in ambulatory surgery. *Nursing Clinics of North America, 32*(2), 441-456.

Lebenbom-Mansour, M.H., Oesterle, J.R., Ownby, D.R., Jennett, M.K., Post, S.K. & Zaflaniczy, K. (1997). The incidence of latex sensitivity in ambulatory surgical patients: A correlation of historical factors with positive serum immunoglobulin E levels. *Anesthesia and Analgesia, 85*(1), 44-49.

Liu, L.L. & Leung, J.M. (2006). *Perioperative complications in elderly patients.* Retrieved April 26, 2009, from http://asahg.org/clinical/geriatrics/perio_comp.htm

Litwack, K. (1997). Care of the special needs patient. *Nursing Clinics of North America, 32*(2), 452-468.

Long, M.C. (1997). Ambulatory anesthesia. In W.E. Hurford, M.T. Bailin, J.K. Davison, K.L. Haspel & C. Rosow (Eds.), *Clinical anesthesia procedures of the Massachusetts General Hospital* (pp. 547-561). Philadelphia: Lippincott-Raven.

Lupien, A.E., Schoneboom, B.A. & Wren, K.R. (2000). Limitations to self-care in the ambulatory surgical patient. *Journal of PeriAnesthesia Nursing, 15*(2), 102-107.

Malignant Hyperthermia Association of the United States. (1999). *Clinical update 1999/00 managing malignant hyperthermia.* Shelburne, NY: Author.

Mamaril, M. (2000). Fast-tracking the postanesthesia patient: The pros and cons. *Journal of PeriAnesthesia Nursing, 15*(2), 89-93.

Manno, M. & Hayes, D.D. (2006). Best-practise interventions: How medication reconciliation saves lives. *Nursing, 36*(3), 63-64.

Martin, J.L. & Njoku, D.B. (2005). Metabolism and toxicity of modern inhaled anesthetics. In Miller, R. (Ed.), *Miller's anesthesia* (6th ed., pp 231-272), Philadelphia: Elsevier Churchill Livingstone.

Martinez, J.B., Moos, D.D. & Dahlen, L.L. (2006). *Journal of PeriAnesthesia Nursing, 21*(2), 82-87.

McCaffery, M. & Beebe, A. (1993). *Pain: Clinical manual for nursing practice.* Baltimore: V.V. Mosby Company.

McCamant, K.L. (2006). Peripheral nerve blocks: Understanding the nurse's role. *Journal of PeriAnesthesia Nursing, 21*(1), 16-26.

McDonald, A. & Leyhane, T. (2005). Drill down with root cause analysis. *Nursing Management, 36*(10), 26-32.

McEwen, D.R. (2003). Ambulatory surgery. In *Alexander's care of the patient in surgery* (12th ed., pp. 1189-1210). St. Louis: Mosby.

McLeskey, C.H. (2006). *Pharmacokinetic and pharmacodynamic differences in the elderly.* Retrieved April 26, 2009, from http://www.asahq.org/clinical/geriatrics/pharma.htm

Mecca, R.S. & Serrins, M.J. (1997). Postanesthesia recovery. In M. Brown & E.M. Brown (Eds.), *Comprehensive postanesthesia care* (pp. 16-36). Baltimore: Williams & Wilkins.

Medicare Payment Advisory Commission. (2004). Report to the congress: Medicare payment policy. Accessed June 11, 2009, from http://www.medpac.gov/documents/Mar04_Entire_report v3.pdf

Meeker, M.H. & Rothrock, J.C. (1999). *Alexander's care of the patient in surgery* (11th ed. pp. 74-75). St. Louis: Mosby.

Merkel, S., Voepel-Lewis, T., Shayevitz, J., & Malviya, S. (1997). The FLACC: A beharioral scale for scoring postoperative pain in young children. *Pediatric Nursing, 23*:293-297.

Messner, R.L. & Lewis, S.J. (1996). *Increasing patient satisfaction: A guide for nurses.* New York: Springer Publishing Co.

Meyer, T.A. (2007). Propofol safety review. *APSF Newsletter, 22*(2).

Mitchell, M. (2004). Pain management in day-case surgery. *Nursing Standard, 18*(25), 33-38.

Monk, T.G. (2004). Anesthesiology's important role in postoperative cognitive impairment research. *ASA Newsletter, 68*(5).

Moos, D.D. & Cuddeford, J.D. (2006). Implications of obstructive sleep apnea syndrome for the perianesthesia. nurse. *Journal of PeriAnesthesia Nursing, 21*(2), 103-118.

Moos, D.D., Prasch, M., Cantral, D.E., Huls, B., & Cuddeford, J.D. (2005). Are patients with obstructive sleep apnea syndrome appropriate for the ambulatory surgical center? *AANA Journal, 73*(3), 197-205.

Morgan, G. E., Mikhail, M. S., & Murray, M.J. (Eds.) 2006. *Clinical anesthesiology* (4th ed.). New York: Mcgraw Hill.

Mulroy, M.F. (2006). Outpatient spinal anesthesia: Is 2-chloroprocaine the answer? *Ambulatory Anesthesia,* April 2006, 50(2),4-5.

Mulroy, F.M. & Owens, B.D. (1997). Postoperative pain management. In M. Brown & E.M. Brown (Eds.), *Comprehensive postanesthesia care* (pp. 89-104). Baltimore: Williams & Wilkins.

Muravchick, S. (2002). Outpatient anesthesia in the geriatric patient. In B.O.Ogunnaike, *Ambulatory Anesthesia, 17*(4), 5.

Muravchick, S. (1997). Geriatric patients. In D.E. Longnecker & F.L. Murphy (Eds.), *Introduction to anesthesia* (9th ed., pp. 364-375). Philadelphia: W.B. Saunders Company.

Murphy, F.L. (1997). Hazards of anesthesia. In D.E. Longnecker & F.L. Murphy (Eds.), *Introduction to anesthesia* (9th ed., pp. 476-484). Philadelphia: W.B. Saunders Company

Nagelhout, J.J. & Boytim, M.J. (2001). Pharmacologic rational for anesthetic agents in ambulatory practice. *Journal of PeriAnesthesia Nursing, 16*(6), 371-378.

Nettina, S.M. (Ed.) (2006). *Lippincott manual of nursing practice* (8th ed.). Philadelphia: Lippincott, Williams & Wilkins.

Noble, K.A. (2005). The patient with latex allergy. *Journal of PeriAnesthesia Nursing, 20*(4), 285-288.

O'Donnell, J.M., Bragg, K. & Sell, S. (2003). Procedural sedation. *Nursing, 33*(4), 36-44.

Olmas, S.R. (2007). Sleep-disordered beathing. *Dental CE Digest, 13*(6),49-52.

Pandit, S.K. (2000). Tea and toast for breakfast before elective surgery? *Ambulatory Anesthesia, 15*(3), 10-11.

Pandit, S.K. (1999). Ambulatory anesthesia and surgery in America: A historical background and recent innovations. *Journal of PeriAnesthesia Nursing, 14*(5), 270-274.

Pape, T.M., Guerra, D.M., Muzquiz, M., Bryant, J., Ingram, M., Schranner, B., et al. (2005). Innovative approaches to reduce nurses' distractions during medication administration. *Journal of Continuing Education in Nursing, 36*(3), 108-116.

Pasero, C. (2005). Fentanyl for acute pain management. *Journal of PeriAnesthesia Nursing, 20*(4), 279-284.

Pasero, C. (2006). Lidocaine iontophoresis for dermal procedure analgesia. *Journal of PeriAnesthesia Nursing, 21*(1), 48-52.

Pasero, C. & Belden, J. (2006). Evidence-based perianesthesia care: Accelerated postoperative Recovery Programs. *Journal of PeriAnesthesia Nursing, 21*(3), 168-76.

Percy, L. (2007). Oregon adopts office-based surgery regulations. *ASA Newsletter, 71*(1).

Plews-Ogan, M.L., Nadkami, M.M., Forren, S., Leon, D., White, D,. Marineau, D., et al. (2004). Patient safety in the ambulatory setting; A clinician based approach, *Journal of General Internal Medicine, 19*(7), 719-25.

Radtke, K. (2004). Get to the root of sentinel events involving infection control. *Nursing Management, 35*(6), 18-22.

Remensnyder, J.P. (1998). Quality issues in ambulatory care. In B.D. Schirmer & D.W. Rattner (Eds.), *Ambulatory surgery* (pp. 49-57). Philadelphia: W.B. Saunders Company.

Reves, J.G., Glass, P., Lubarsky, D., & McEvoy, M. (2005). Intravenous nonopiod anesthetics. In R. Miller (Ed.), *Miller's anesthesia* (6th ed.). Philadelphia: Elsevier Churchill Livingstone.

Riley, G.P. (2003). Intravenous conscious sedation: "Pearls and perils." Armed Forces Institute of Pathology, Nursing Risk Management 2003.

Roberge, C.W. & McEwen, M. (1998). The effects of local anesthetics on postoperative pain. *AORN Journal, 68*(6), 1003-101.

Rosenberg, H. & Kaplan. R.F. (2006). Malignant hyperthermia in the ambulatory setting. *Ambulatory Anesthesia, 21*(1), 4-5.

Rosenberg, H. & Rothstein, A. (2006). Malignant hyperthermia death holds many lessons. APSF Newsletter. *Journal of the Anesthesia Patient Safety Foundation, 21*(1), 32-34.

Rothrock, J.C. (Ed.) (2003). *Alexander's care of the patient in surgery* (12th ed.). St. Louis: Mosby.

Rozner, M.A. (2006). Informing the misinformed about ICDs. *ASA Newsletter, 70*(1).

Saufl, N.M. (2006). Reconciliation of medications. *Journal of PeriAnesthesia Nursing, 21*(2), 126-127

Scanlon, J. & Richards, B. (2004). Development of a same day laminectomy program. *Journal of PeriAnesthesia Nursing, 19*(2), 84-86.

Scher, C.S. (1998, October). Widespread psychiatric drug use points to need to explore interactions with anesthesia. Paper presented at the annual meeting of the American Society of Anesthesiologists, Orlando, FL.

Schirmer, B.D. & Rattner, D.W. (Eds.) (1998). *Ambulatory surgery* (pp. 181-190). Philadelphia: W.B. Saunders Company.

Semo, J.J. (2005). Propofol sedation by nonanesthesiologists: A medicolegal gamble? *Ambulatory Anesthesia, 20*(1), 3-5.

Shankar, V. & Deshpand, J.K. (2005). Procedural sedation in the pediatric patient. *Anesthesiology Clinics of North America, 23,* 633-654.

Shumaker, R.P. (1997). Perioperative nursing. In J.M. Black & E. Matassarian-Jacobs (Eds.), *Medical-surgical nursing: Clinical management for continuity of care* (5th ed., pp. 449-493). Philadelphia: W.B. Saunders Company.

Sieber, F. & Pauldine, R. (2005). Anesthesia for the elderly. In R. Miller (Ed.), *Miller's anesthesia* (6th ed.). Philadelphia: Elsevier Churchill Livingstone.

Small, S.D. (1998). Special considerations for laparoscopic surgery. In B.D. Schirmer & D.W. Rattner (Eds.), *Ambulatory surgery* (pp. 181-190). Philadelphia: W.B. Saunders Company.

Smith, M.S, Muir, H., & Hall, R. (1996). Preoperative management of drug therapy: Clinical considerations. *Drugs, 51,* 238-259.

SurgiStrategies. (2006, February). *Parents happier with alternative to liquid meds for tonsillectomy.* Retrieved April 26, 2009, from http://www.surgicenteronline.com/hotnews/62h18584820742.html

Stone, D.J. & Gal, T.J. (2005). Airway management. In R. Miller (Ed.), *Miller's anesthesia* (6th ed., pp. 1414-1451), Philadelphia: Elsevier Churchill Livingstone.

Sutton, G.P., Rodgers, R.E., Hurd, W.W., & Mutone, M.F. (2005). Gynecology. In F.C. Brunicardi, D.K. Anderson, T.R. Billiar, D.L. Dunn, J.G. Hunter, & R.G. Pollack (Eds.), *Schwartz's principles of surgery* (8th ed.). New York: McGraw Hill, Health Publishing Division.

Sweitzer, B.J. (1998). Conscious sedation. In B.D. Schirmer & D.W. Rattner (Eds.), *Ambulatory surgery* (pp. 137-150). Philadelphia: W.B. Saunders Company.

Tarrac, S.E. (2006). A description of intraoperative and postanesthesia complication rates. *Journal of PeriAnesthesia Nursing, 21*(2), 88-96.

Tang, J., Wang, B., White, P.F., Watcha, M.F., Qi, J., & Wender, R.H. (1998). The effect of timing of ondansetron administration on its efficacy, cost-effectiveness, and cost-benefit as a prophylactic antiemetic in the ambulatory setting. *Anesthesia & Analgesia, 86*(2), 274-282.

Terris, D.J., Moister, B., Seybt, M., Gourin, G., & Chin, E. (2006). Study indicates outpatient thyroid surgery is safe and desirable. Presented at the 110th Annual Meeting, the American Academy of Otolaryngology, Toronto, Canada.

Tesniere, A. & Servin, F. (2003). *Anesthesiology Clinics of North America, 21,* 273-288.

Tetzlaff, J.E. (1996). Peripheral nerve blocks. In G.E. Morgan & M.S. Mikhail (Eds.), *Clinical anesthesiology* (2nd ed., pp. 245-273). Stamford: Appleton & Lange.

The Joint Commission. (2009, October 21). *2009 national patient safety goals ambulatory care program.* Retrieved April 25, 2009, from http://www.jointcommission.org/PatientSafety/NationalPatientSafetyGoals/09_amb_npsgs.htm

The Joint Commission. (2009). "Do not use list." Retrieved June 11, 2009, from http://www.jointcommission.org/PatientSafety/DoNotUseList/

The Joint Commission. (2007). *Sentinel event policy and procedures.* Retrieved June 11, 2009, from http://www.jointcommission.org/SentinelEvents/PolicyandProcedures/

The Joint Commission Resources. (2006a). Joint Commission perspectives on patient safety: Applying aviation principles to health care. 6(1), 7-9.

The Joint Commission Resources. (2006b). Joint Commission perspectives on patient safety: Civility in the health care workplace. 6(1), 1-3.

The Joint Commission. (2004). *Sentinel event alert: Preventing, and managing the impact of, anesthesia awareness.* Issue 32. Retrieved April 26, 2009, from http://www.jointcommission.org/SentinelEvents/SentinelEventAlert/sea_32.htm

Verghese, S.T. & Hannallah, R.S. (2005). Postoperative pain management in children, *Anesthesiology Clinics of North America, 23,* 163-184.

Vira, T., Colquhoun, M., & Etchells, E. (2006). Reconcilable differences: Correcting medication errors at hospital admission and discharge. *Quality and Safetynin Health Care, 15*(2), 122-126.

Viby-Mogensen, J. (2005). Neuromuscular monitoring. In R. Miller (Ed.), *Miller's anesthesia* (6th ed., pp. 1351-1366). Philadelphia: Elsevier Churchill Livingstone.

Vitkun, S.A. (1997). Allergic reactions. In M. Brown & E.M. Brown (Eds.), *Comprehensive postanesthesia care* (pp. 347-380). Baltimore: Williams & Wilkins.

Wadlund, D.L. (2006). Laparoscopy: Risks, benefits and complications. *Nursing Clinics of North America, 41,* 219-229.

Watkins, A.C. & White, P.F. (2001). Fast-tracking after ambulatory surgery. *Journal of Peri Anesthesia Nursing, 16*(6), 379-387.

Watt-Watson, J., Chung, F., Chan, V.W.S., & McGillion, M. (2004). Pain management following discharge after ambulatory same-day surgery. *Journal of Nursing Management, 12,* 153-164.

Wedel, D.J. & Horlacher, T.T. (2005). Nerve blocks. In R. Miller (Ed.), *Miller's anesthesia* (6th ed., pp. 1685-1718). Philadelphia: Elsevier Churchill Livingstone.

White, J.L. & Durieux, M.E. (2005). Clinical pharmacology of local anesthetics. *Anesthesiology Clinics of North America, 23*(1).

White, P.F. & Recart-Friere, A. (2005). Ambulatory (outpatient) anesthesia. In R. Miller (Ed.), *Miller's anesthesia* (6th ed., pp. 2589-2635). Philadelphia: Elsevier Churchill Livingstone.

Winslow, E.H. & Jacobson, A.F. (1997). Preop fluid bolus reduces adverse surgical effects. *American Journal of Nursing, 97*(3), 62.

Yemen, T.A. (1998). Managing the pediatric outpatient. In B.D. Schirmer & D.W. Rattner (Eds.), *Ambulatory surgery* (pp. 167-180). Philadelphia: W.B. Saunders Company.

Yellen, E. (2003). The influence of nurse-sensitive variables on patient satisfaction. *AORN 78*(5), 783-793.

Zanchetta, C. & Bernstein, M. (2004). The nursing role in patient education regarding outpatient neurosurgical procedures. *AXON, 25*(4), 18-21.

Zwass, M.S. (2005). Regional anesthesia in children. *Anesthesiology Clinics of North America, 23,* 815-835.

INDEX

Page references followed by *fig* indicate an illustrated figure; followed by *t* indicate a table.

P